Healthy Living
with

high FIBRE

Murdoch Books Australia
Pier 8/9
23 Hickson Road
Millers Point NSW 2000
Phone: +61 (0) 2 8220 2000
Fax: +61 (0) 2 8220 2558

Murdoch Books UK Limited
Erico House
6th Floor North
93–99 Upper Richmond Road
Putney, London SW15 2TG
Phone: +44 (0) 20 8785 5995
Fax: +44 (0) 20 8785 5985

Published in 2011 by Murdoch Books Pty Limited
www.murdochbooks.com.au

For Corporate Orders & Custom Publishing contact Noel Hammond, National Business Development Manager

Publisher: Lynn Lewis
Designer: Jacqueline Richards
Food Consultants: Jayne Tancred and Toni Gumley
Photographer: Ian Hofstetter
Stylists: Jane Collins and Katy Holder
Food preparation: Joanne Kelly and Grace Campbell
Recipes by: Michelle Earl and members of the Murdoch Books Test Kitchen
Project Editor: Alice Grundy
Production: Joan Beal

National Library of Australia Cataloguing-in-Publication entry
Title: Healthy living: high fibre.
ISBN: 9781742668888 (pbk.)
Notes: Includes index.
Subjects: Cooking.
High-fibre diet--Recipes. Fibre in human nutrition.
Dewey Number: 641.5637

A catalogue record for this book is available from the British Library.

PRINTED IN CHINA.

IMPORTANT: Those who might be at risk from the effects of salmonella poisoning (the elderly, pregnant women, young children and those suffering from immune deficiency diseases) should consult their doctor with any concerns about eating raw eggs.

OVEN GUIDE: You may find cooking times vary depending on the oven you are using. For fan-forced ovens, as a general rule, set the oven temperature to 20°C (35°F) lower than indicated in the recipe.

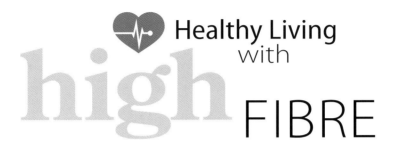

Healthy Living
with
high FIBRE

EASY *high-fibre*
RECIPES AND LIFESTYLE SOLUTIONS

Introductory text by Dr Susanna Holt (PhD, Dietitian)

MURDOCH BOOKS

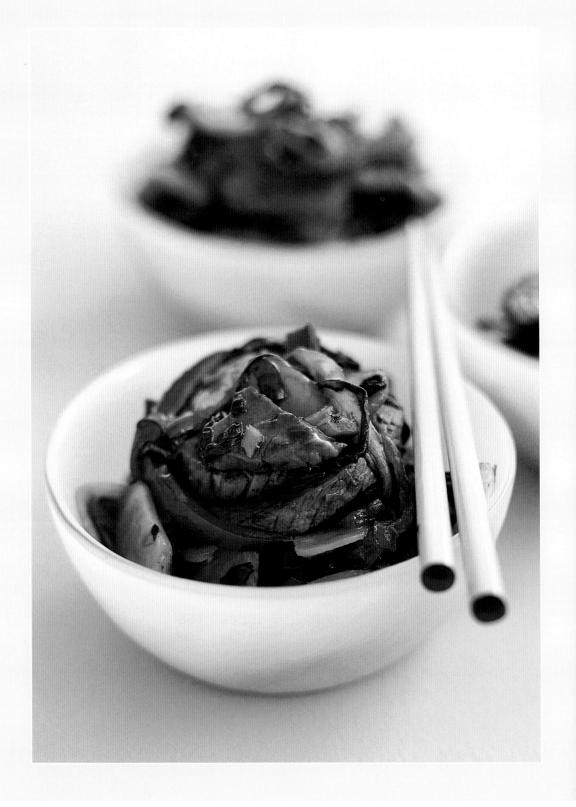

contents

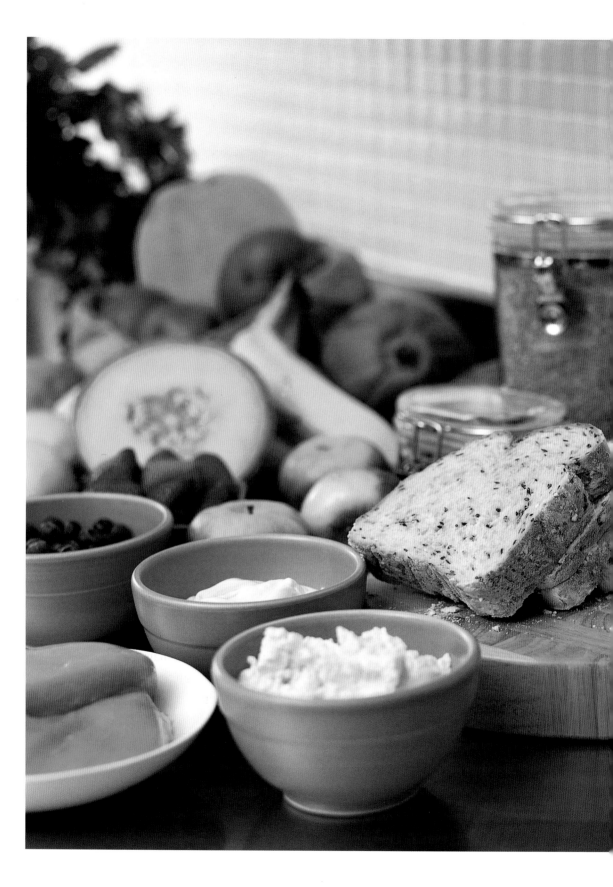

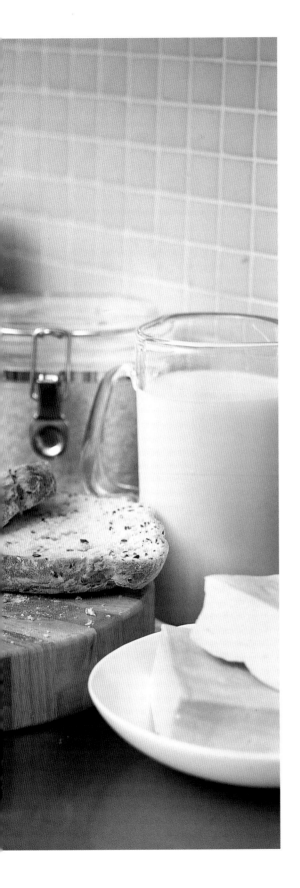

Good health
WITH
high
FIBRE

You know fibre helps keep your digestive system healthy, but are you aware of how many other benefits high-fibre diets have to offer? A fibre-rich diet may help control your weight, blood sugar and cholesterol levels, and reduce your risk of developing heart disease, type 2 diabetes and certain types of cancer.

Health surveys show that most people in industrialised countries don't eat enough fibre on a regular basis for good long-term health. You may find this surprising after you read the following pages and learn how easy it is to add more fibre to your daily diet.

Despite ongoing health campaigns that try to educate people about the importance of a nutritious diet, dietary surveys continue to show that many people regularly eat less than the recommended amounts of fruit, vegetables, wholegrain products and legumes.

The good news is that simply by changing your eating habits to include more fibre-rich foods and less fat and overly processed foods in your diet, you can achieve a lot of healthy eating goals at the same time—you will increase your intake of fibre and healthy antioxidants while decreasing your intake of saturated fat.

A healthier diet together with regular exercise will help make you look good and feel good, and will reduce your risk of weight gain and the diseases that many people develop as they get older, such as high blood pressure, high blood cholesterol, haemorrhoids and diabetes. By being well nourished and active, you'll also find it easier to perform both mental and physical tasks, which helps make them more enjoyable.

Fibre—the natural laxative

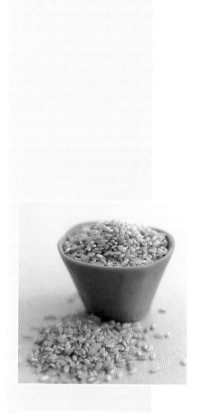

Studies have shown that a high intake of fibre from wholegrain cereal foods, such as natural muesli, wholegrain bread and brown rice, is associated with a lower risk of digestive tract cancers (including stomach and bowel cancer). Given all of fibre's health properties, it's a shame that we don't include more of this natural laxative in our daily diets.

Oral laxatives, sold over the counter, are amongst the top-selling pharmaceutical products in industrialised countries around the world. Regular laxative use should be avoided because you may need ever-increasing doses to achieve the desired effect, which increases the risk of other health problems. Many people would not need to use laxatives if they simply increased their fibre and water intake and did more physical activity.

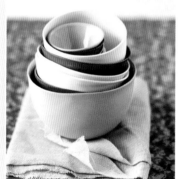

How can this book help you?

It's not hard to improve your diet and lifestyle, you just need to get organised. Schedule regular exercise into your weekly activities and keep your refrigerator and pantry well stocked with healthy foods.

This book will help by providing information about the health-promoting properties of a fibre-rich diet along with practical advice so you can easily increase your fibre intake. It contains a variety of tested recipes that provide good amounts of fibre while also meeting other healthy eating guidelines, such as being lower in fat.

Health surveys show that most people in industrialised countries don't eat enough fibre on a regular basis for good long-term health.

Most of the recipes in this book provide at least 5–6 grams of fibre per serve; a few of the baking recipes contain less than 5 grams of fibre per serve, but more than is found in the regular version of the recipe. Among the recipes, you'll find options for healthy, everyday meals that the whole family will enjoy, as well as dishes that can be prepared for special occasions.

It's never too late to start roughing it. Increase your fibre intake and reap the health benefits of a high-fibre diet based on fruits, vegetables, legumes and grain products.

What is fibre?

Dietary fibre, also known as roughage, is found in plant foods, such as grains, nuts, seeds, legumes, fruit, vegetables and seaweed. Animal foods such as meat, fish, chicken, eggs and cow's milk do not contain any fibre.

Fibre refers to any component of plant foods that cannot be digested (broken down) by human digestive enzymes. The fibrous strings in celery and green beans, and the white pithy membrane of citrus fruit are visible examples of fibre.

Other than lignin, the different types of fibre are all types of carbohydrate because they are made up of chains of individual sugar units bound together. However, your digestive enzymes cannot break down the sugar chains in fibre in the same way they break down the sugar chains in other dietary carbohydrates (sugars and starches), so fibre remains undigested as it passes through your stomach and small intestine and moves down to the lower intestine.

Different types of dietary fibre have different effects in the body due to variations in their chemical structure.

Different types of fibre

Plant foods typically contain a mixture of the two main types of dietary fibre: insoluble and soluble fibre. Resistant starch and non-digestible oligosaccharides are two other types of indigestible carbohydrates found in plant foods, and are classified as fibre by scientists due to their fibre-like effects in the body.

Different types of dietary fibre have different effects in the body due to variations in their chemical structure.

Insoluble fibre doesn't dissolve in water, but can soak up a lot of water inside your stomach and intestines. The indigestible fibre and extra water increases the bulk of the food contents, which helps push the digested food matter through your digestive system, removing waste materials and preventing constipation. You can think of it as a natural laxative that, together with water, helps flush out your system.

The compounds in food that are classified as insoluble fibre include cellulose, hemicellulose and lignin, which make up the structural parts of plant cell walls. Good sources include wholegrain bread, brown rice, wheat bran, rice bran, nuts, seeds, legumes and unpeeled fruit and vegetables.

Soluble fibre absorbs water or partially dissolves in water. It forms a gel-like substance in the stomach and intestines, and if enough of it is consumed at a meal it can help slow down the rate of food digestion and reduce the extent to which your blood sugar level rises as you digest your food.

As with insoluble fibre, the water absorbed by soluble fibre adds bulk to food contents and helps push them through your digestive system. However, soluble fibre is different from insoluble fibre in that the 'friendly' bacteria that live in your intestine can ferment it. The fatty acids that are produced during the fermentation process provide the bacteria with a source of energy and also produce some beneficial effects in your body, including supporting your immunity and helping to reduce your risk of heart disease and bowel cancer.

The compounds in food that are classified as soluble fibre include pectins, gums and mucilage, which are mainly found around and inside plant cells. Good sources include oat bran, psyllium fibre, linseeds (flax seeds), barley and legumes such as chickpeas and cannellini beans. Due to their gelling effects, soluble fibres like pectins and gums are also sometimes added to processed foods such as jams and sauces, where they act as thickening or setting agents.

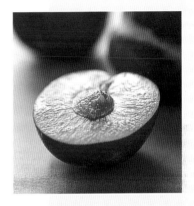

Resistant starch is starch (a type of carbohydrate) that isn't digested in the small intestine and instead passes into the large intestine. It doesn't absorb lots of water like soluble and insoluble fibre do, so it doesn't increase the bulk of food matter in your gut. However, like soluble fibre, it can be fermented by the bacteria that live in your large intestine, and therefore has some health benefits.

The reason some resistant starch can't be digested is that it's physically trapped in foods where your digestive enzymes can't reach it, for example, inside seeds, lentils and whole grains. Some resistant starch is formed in starchy foods after they have been cooked and subsequently cooled down. For example, in bread, cold cooked potatoes (cold potato salad), rice (sushi) and pasta (pasta salad). Resistant starch (for example, Hi-Maize) is also sometimes added to processed foods such as white bread, snack bars and breakfast cereals to increase their 'fibre' content.

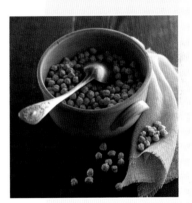

Non-digestible oligosaccharides are small carbohydrates (bigger than a sugar but smaller than a starch) that cannot be digested by enzymes in the human stomach or small intestine. Like soluble fibre and resistant starch, they pass undigested into the large intestine where they are fermented by bacteria, resulting in the production of gas and fatty acids. (This is one reason some people experience gas after they eat legumes.)

Oligosaccharides include raffinose, inulin, stachyose and oligofructose. They are found in legumes and certain vegetables (such as artichokes, leeks, onions and garlic). Inulin is also found in some processed foods, such as some yoghurts, where it's added as a prebiotic to help stimulate the growth of beneficial bacteria.

Fibre and Your Health

How does fibre help keep your digestive system healthy?

The human digestive system is a very efficient system that we tend to take for granted until something goes wrong. Many people in industrialised countries eat a low-fibre diet and consequently develop gastrointestinal problems as they age, such as chronic constipation, haemorrhoids, diverticular disease and colon (bowel) cancer. A high-fibre diet helps speed up the process of food elimination, and is an easy way to help protect your digestive system from future problems.

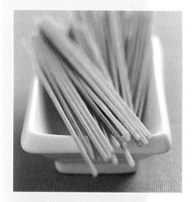

After you eat a meal, insoluble and soluble fibre in the food absorbs and binds a lot of water. As a result the food matter becomes larger, softer and bulkier. The increased bulk stimulates the process of peristalsis, in which muscular contractions push the digested food down towards the lower (large) intestine. This process occurs more quickly and easily with a high-fibre diet.

Low-fibre meals soak up less water in your gastrointestinal tract, so stools comprised of low-fibre food waste tend to be smaller and harder. They take longer to move through the digestive system, and are more difficult to pass from the body. (The slowing down effect of soluble fibre on food digestion tends to be overridden by the bulking effect of insoluble fibre, unless a large amount of soluble fibre is eaten. Most meals contain more insoluble fibre than soluble fibre.)

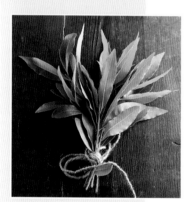

Countering Constipation

Constipation is defined as having fewer than three bowel movements a week. However, normal stool elimination can vary from three times a day to three times a week, and some people feel constipated if they don't have at least one bowel movement a day.

Typically, constipation occurs when the muscular contractions of the large intestine are slow or sluggish, causing the stool to move too slowly. As a result, the stool becomes hard and dry and more difficult to eliminate.

Constipation is a common problem in industrialised societies and especially so among older people. It is typically caused by a low-fibre diet, a lack of physical activity, dehydration and/or poor

A high-fibre diet helps speed up the process of food elimination, and is an easy way to help protect your digestive system from future problems.

fluid consumption. The presence of certain health problems or the use of certain medications (including the overuse of laxatives) may also be involved.

It's important to avoid chronic constipation because it can lead to complications such as haemorrhoids, anal tears or a rectal prolapse due to the increased strain required for bowel movements.

See your doctor for advice if you regularly suffer from constipation. You could also see a dietitian for advice about how you can gradually increase your fibre intake.

In most cases you can prevent or treat constipation by increasing your fibre consumption to 20–35 grams a day, drinking more water (ideally eight glasses per day) and increasing your physical activity.

Diverticular disease

After the age of 40, many people develop diverticula, which are small pouches that bulge out of the inner part of the colon (like an inner tube that pokes out of a weak spot in a bicycle tyre). This condition is called diverticulosis or diverticular disease. In around 10-25 percent of people with diverticula, the pouches become inflamed or infected, a condition called diverticulosis.

Many people with diverticular disease do not have any discomfort, but others experience cramps, abdominal bloating and constipation. Stress, medications and other health disorders, such as irritable bowel syndrome (IBS), can cause similar symptoms, so it's important to see your doctor if you regularly experience these symptoms.

Diverticular disease can lead to complications such as infections, tears or a blockage that requires surgery. The most common cause of diverticular disease is thought to be constipation resulting from a low-fibre, high-fat diet. Constipation makes it much harder to pass a stool, and the increased pressure could cause weak spots in the colon to bulge out and form diverticula.

Diverticular disease and constipation are rare among rural communities in less-developed countries where people are very active and eat high-fibre diets.

A high-fibre diet (and sometimes a fibre supplement) along with plenty of water is the only treatment required by most people with diverticular disease. In some cases, antibiotics and/or pain-relieving medicines are prescribed for acute flare-ups of diverticulitis.

Irritable bowel syndrome

Irritable bowel syndrome (IBS) is classified as a functional bowel disorder - a condition that does not appear to be due to any physical abnormalities. Symptoms vary from person to person, but it tends to be characterised by abdominal pain, gas, bloating and cramps with constipation and/or diarrhoea.

See your doctor for an assessment if you've experienced abdominal pain or discomfort, diarrhoea and/or constipation, over at least 12 weeks of the past year (not necessarily consecutively). These symptoms could be due to IBS or a number of other bowel conditions (including lactose intolerance or coeliac disease). It's important to get an accurate diagnosis so you can start the proper treatment as soon as possible.

No clear cause of IBS has been established. However, possible causes include problems with the bowel's muscular contractions due to illness, infection or some psychological factors such as prolonged stress.

Certain dietary factors may also be involved, and there are a number of dietary changes a person with IBS can make to reduce pain, discomfort and bowel problems, however a wide degree of individual variation occurs, and not all dietary changes lead to improved symptoms in all sufferers.

You may need to record your responses to different foods in a diary, and then work with your doctor or dietitian to arrive at an optimal dietary plan for your personal circumstances. The best diet for you may depend on your prevailing symptoms at a given time.

In general, some people with IBS find it helpful to avoid or cut back on:

- Foods rich in insoluble fibre, such as bran cereals, legumes and unpeeled vegetables (especially when diarrhoea or cramping are present)
- Eating large meals
- Oily foods
- Dairy foods (even when there is no lactose intolerance)
- Coffee, alcohol, cola and other carbonated drinks
- Chocolate
- Chewing gum

Instead, try the following:

- Foods rich in soluble fibre (which may help to relieve constipation), such as fruit, vegetables and oats
- Eating frequent, small meals
- Water (especially important if you're suffering from diarrhoea, which may lead to dehydration)

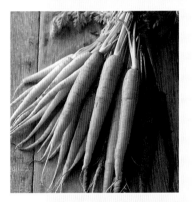

Additionally, research suggests that some people with IBS may benefit from adopting a diet that's low in certain chemicals that are naturally present in foods. These compounds include fermentable oligosaccharides, disaccharides, monosaccharides and polyols, and are collectively referred to as FODMAPs. To determine whether a low-FODMAP diet may be appropriate for your circumstances, talk to your doctor or dietitian.

Colon (bowel) cancer

A number of scientific studies have shown that eating a diet that's low in fat and rich in wholegrain foods has a protective effect against cancer, and particularly cancer of the colon (the lower half of your bowel).

Several factors are believed to contribute to this effect. For example, high-fibre foods like wholegrains speed up the movement of food matter through the colon, which reduces the amount of time your colon is in contact with any cancer-promoting chemicals in the faecal contents. Besides fibre, other compounds present in wholegrains are also believed to be involved, including the fermentable oligosaccharides that provide an energy source for the friendly bacteria in the bowel. It's also possible that the effects are at least partially due to the reduced levels of insulin and/or

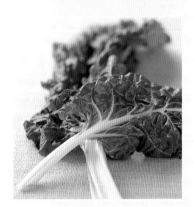

inflammation that result from this way of eating.

On the other hand, people who eat low fibre diets and an excess of fatty food are at increased risk of developing colonic polyps. These are abnormal tissue growths that occur in the mucous membrane of the colon. While some polyps are benign (not dangerous) others are cancerous or precancerous. Most polyps don't cause any symptoms, so they are usually only discovered when doctors perform routine colon cancer screening tests (such as a rectal examination or a colonoscopy).

How does fibre help with weight control?

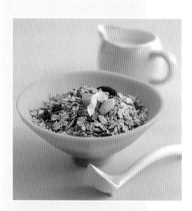

Many overweight people find it easier to lose weight when their diet is modified to include more healthy foods with less fat and more fibre.

Think about how easy it is to drink a glass of apple juice, but how difficult it would be to eat three whole apples in the same amount of time. Although you're consuming roughly the same amount of kilojoules, the whole apples make you full much faster than the juice, simply because your jaws have to work much harder to chew and swallow the larger volume of whole apples. This slows down the speed at which you eat, giving your brain time to register the growing feeling of fullness in your stomach.

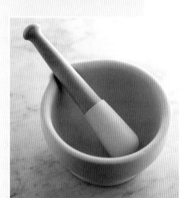

You may not even be able to eat three apples in one go, but you could easily drink them in a glass of juice. Unlike the whole apples that still contain their fibre intact, the fibre in the apple juice has been ground up into smaller particles by the juicing process. The ground-up fibre is less effective in your body because it is less able to bind water and increase the bulk of your stomach contents.

Just like the apples, cereal grains such as wheat become easier to eat and less filling as they are progressively ground down from whole grains into cracked grains, then into coarse flour and then fine flour. They also become more easily digested, which increases their effects on your blood sugar and insulin levels.

Bread made from fine wheat flour has a higher blood sugar-raising effect (high glycaemic index, or GI value) than bread made from coarsely ground flour or bread with whole grains in it. Consequently, the fibre content on a food label may not always be a good indication of how 'healthy' that fibre is. Some brands of wholemeal (whole-wheat) bread have a similar fibre content to

Many overweight people find it easier to lose weight when their diet is modified to include more healthy foods with less fat and more fibre.

some grainy breads, but their fibre has a finer texture and is not as effective as the fibre in the wholegrain bread. Similarly, some types of wholegrain bread have more fibre in them than other varieties. Look for wholegrain bread with lots of visible grains in it; the more grains you can see, the more intact fibre is present.

Plant foods are more filling and useful for weight control when they're less processed and closer to their natural state (for example, brown rice instead of white rice, wholegrain bread instead of white or wholemeal bread). Foods with intact or relatively unprocessed fibre are more difficult to chew and swallow, which helps slow down your eating rate and makes it easier for you to realise when you're starting to feel full. The nerves and muscles that are activated while you chew and swallow foods send signals to your brain to stimulate the sensation of fullness.

This way, it's possible to eat filling, satisfying meals and still keep your weight in check. You just need to make smarter food choices focusing on both the type and amount of food you eat. Eat unpeeled fruit and vegetables, and choose brown rice and wholegrain bread. Don't mash your potatoes; instead eat them whole in their skin as baked potatoes. Eat fruit instead of drinking it, and when time permits, boil legumes instead of tinned ones, which are softer.

Choosing foods that are harder to chew and swallow can make it harder for you to overeat, making weight control easier.

How can fibre aid diabetes?

A high-fibre diet can help reduce your risk of developing type 2 diabetes or help you control your blood sugar if you have the condition.

Soluble fibre in food can form a viscous gel when mixed with fluid in the digestive tract. This makes it harder for digestive enzymes to reach the food particles, which slows down the rate of

A lower fat, high-fibre diet based on plant foods plus regular exercise reduces the risk of developing type 2 diabetes as you get older.

As part of a healthy diet and lifestyle, eating low-GI foods has many health benefits to offer those with diabetes or pre-diabetes: lower blood cholesterol, a lower risk of heart problems, and blood glucose and diabetes can be better managed. A low-GI diet can also support your weight loss efforts and improve your sensitivity to insulin.

carbohydrate digestion and results in a slower, more steady release of sugar (glucose) into your bloodstream after a meal.

A lower fat, high-fibre diet based on plant foods plus regular exercise reduces the risk of developing type 2 diabetes as you get older. Further protection can be obtained if you favour carbohydrate-containing foods that have a low glycaemic index (GI, i.e. those that are converted into glucose slowly after you've consumed them) along with healthier sources of dietary fat (monounsaturated and omega-3 polyunsaturated fats).

A healthy diet and active lifestyle make your tissues more sensitive to the effects of insulin, so your body doesn't have to produce as much insulin in order to process the foods you eat. In contrast, a high-fat, high-GI, low-fibre diet requires more insulin to be metabolised, which increases the risk of weight gain, insulin resistance and type 2 diabetes.

Achieving a lower GI diet is easy using the table of lower and higher GI foods on page 23. Start gradually by making one high-for-low GI food swap each day, and over time, increase the number of foods you swap to one at each meal or snack.

If you have diabetes, and especially if you need tablets or insulin, the advice of a dietitian is essential. A dietitian can help you work out the type of eating plan best suited to your health, medication and lifestyle needs.

How does fibre reduce the risk of heart disease?

There is powerful evidence to suggest that a high-fibre diet reduces the risk of heart disease, an effect that is largely attributed to fibre's ability to lower cholesterol, but which may also involve the lower intake of fat and the higher intake of vitamins, minerals, antioxidants and phytochemicals that occurs when people eat more fruit, vegetables, legumes and wholegrain products.

Not all types of fibre have the ability to lower cholesterol. For example, wholemeal wheat products and wheat bran appear to have no effect on serum cholesterol levels. On the other hand, when taken in adequate quantities over a sufficient timeframe, soluble fibre from pectin, oat bran and other wholemeal oat products, psyllium, and several different types of gum have been scientifically proven to lower both total cholesterol and LDL-cholesterol (sometimes referred to as 'bad' cholesterol).

This effect is thought to be largely due to soluble fibre binding to dietary cholesterol and bile acids in the digestive tract and being excreted with the faeces rather than being absorbed by the body. This in turn means the liver needs to use cholesterol from the bloodstream to make new bile acids to replace those that have been lost, resulting in an overall decrease in blood cholesterol levels.

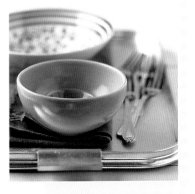

How much fibre should I be eating?

Dietary surveys indicate that most people eat less than 20 grams per day due to inadequate consumption of fruit, vegetables, wholegrain products and legumes.

Australian and New Zealand health authorities advise that an adequate intake of dietary fibre is 30 grams per day for healthy adult men, and 25 grams for healthy adult women, from a variety of foods. However, they recommend 38 grams per day for men, and 28 grams for women for optimal prevention of chronic health problems such as cardiovascular disease, diabetes and some types of cancer. Other countries have similar targets, so aim for a minimum of 25–30 grams per day.

Due to their smaller size and appetites, children need less fibre than adults.

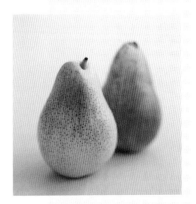

Adequate intake of fibre for children and adolescents

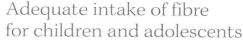

Age group	Boys	Girls
1-3 years	14 g/day	14 g/day
4-8 years	18 g/day	18 g/day
9-13 years	24 g/day	20 g/day
14-18 years	28 g/day	22 g/day

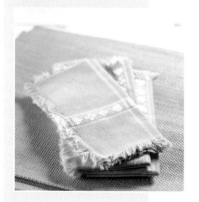

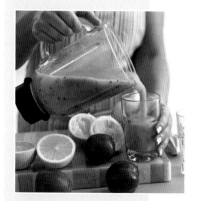

What's the best way to increase my fibre intake?

Eating more fibre is easy because fibre is found in so many foods. All you need to do is follow the general healthy eating guidelines for your age group that are recommended by health authorities, and make your diet more natural by eating mostly fruit, vegetables, grain foods and legumes. This means that most of the food you eat each day should come from these four food groups.

You can then add moderate amounts of lower fat protein-rich foods (lower fat dairy products or alternatives, eggs, lean meat and poultry, fish and seafood) and small amounts of fat (oils, margarine, avocados, olives, sauces, seeds, nuts and dressings).

This way of eating will increase your intake of fibre, antioxidants and phytochemicals while decreasing your intake of saturated fat, salt and added sugars.

See a dietitian if you need help working out the types and amounts of foods you should be eating each day, but in general, each day you should aim to eat:

- At least 5 serves of vegetables (including legumes, which should be eaten at least twice per week); and
- At least two serves of fruit; and
- 4-5 serves of grain-based foods, preferably from wholegrain sources.

Don't forget to drink 8 glasses of water each day too.

How much is a serve?

Food group	Examples of serving sizes
Vegetables	1 cup of fresh salad; or ½ cup of cooked vegetables; or 1 potato
Legumes	½ cup cooked legumes
Fruit	1 medium-sized piece of fruit; or 2 small-sized pieces of fruit; or 1 cup of fresh or canned fruit pieces; or ½ cup of fruit juice; or 1½ tablespoons dried fruit
Grains	2 slices of bread; or 1 medium-sized bread roll; or 1 cup cooked rice, pasta or noodles; or 1 cup cooked porridge; or 1⅓ cups of breakfast cereal; or ½ cup natural muesli
Nuts and seeds	⅓ cup peanuts or almonds; or ¼ cup sunflower or sesame seeds

Changing over to a high-fibre diet

If your fibre intake has previously been low, it's best to increase your fibre and water intake gradually. This will give your digestive system time to adapt and help you avoid any uncomfortable abdominal problems, such as bloating and excess gas, which can sometimes occur if you suddenly start eating high-fibre meals.

If you and your family normally eat white bread, start by switching to wholegrain bread that's not too dense. After a while, you can start buying even grainier breads. There are plenty of delicious grainy breads with different seeds and grains in them that will appeal to different family members. Similarly, if you find it hard to eat a whole bowl of bran or natural muesli, first try eating half a bowl topped with another cereal and some fresh fruit.

It's very important to include high-fibre foods in children's diets, because the extra chewing helps their teeth and jaws develop properly, and also teaches them to appreciate more nutritious foods. Children who are brought up on soft white bread and soft peeled fruits often find it difficult to enjoy grainy bread and unpeeled fruit as they get older, so over the long term they can miss out on the health benefits these foods have to offer.

For children, choosing higher fibre breakfast cereals may be particularly important, and could even help their schooling! In scientific research, school children that ate a low-GI, high-fibre cereal for breakfast (oatmeal) experienced better mental performance and improved memory function than children who ate a low fibre ready-to-eat cereal, or no breakfast at all.

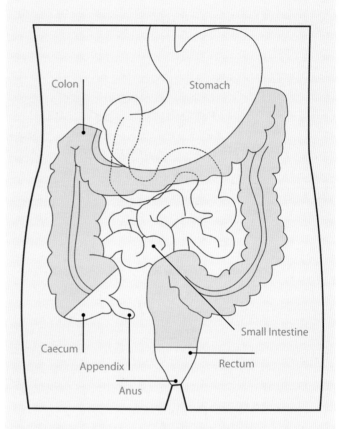

Small intestine and large intestine/colon (shaded)

Healthy eating and lifestyle guidelines

- Eat a variety of nutritious foods each day.
- Base your diet on vegetables, fruit, legumes and grain products (mostly wholegrain and low-GI).
- Eat a variety of different coloured fruits and vegetables each week.
- Eat a lower fat diet with a low saturated fat content.
- Drink alcohol in moderation, if at all.
- Limit your intake of salt and added sugars.
- Regularly eat foods that contain iron and calcium.
- Maintain a healthy weight and be physically active.
- Drink plenty of water each day.

Health benefits of a high-fibre diet

- ○ Prevents constipation, haemorrhoids and diverticular disease
- ○ Increases the number of 'friendly' bacteria in the colon
- ○ Lowers the risk of colon cancer and some other forms of cancer
- ○ Makes weight control easier
- ○ Helps control your blood sugar and cholesterol levels
- ○ Reduces the risk of type 2 diabetes and heart disease

High versus low GI

Type of food	Higher GI Versions	Lower GI Alternatives
Bread	Regular soft textured white, wholemeal or rye bread and bread rolls, white or wholemeal bagels, gluten-free bread, Lebanese bread, melba toast, scones	Wholegrain breads with a relatively dense texture, pumpernickel bread, pita bread, sourdough bread, breads made from coarse stone-ground flour
Grains	Most types of rice (especially jasmine), millet, polenta (cornmeal)	Basmati rice, doongara rice, pearled barley, quinoa, buckwheat, bulgur (cracked wheat)
Pasta and noodles	Gluten-free corn or rice pasta, low-fat instant noodles, dried rice noodles, udon noodles, couscous	Durum wheat pasta—regular or protein-enriched, gluten-free legume-based pasta, mung bean noodles, fresh rice noodles, soba noodles, tortellini, ravioli
Breakfast cereals	Most processed breakfast cereals, including puffed grains (rice, amaranth, wheat, buckwheat), instant porridge, regular wheat breakfast biscuit cereals	Semolina, porridge made from whole or steel-cut oats, oat bran, natural muesli (without flakes), oat bran wheat biscuits
Biscuits and crackers	Puffed crispbreads, water biscuits, wafer biscuits, plain sweet biscuits, morning coffee biscuits	Biscuits (cookies) made with stone-ground flour, whole rolled oats or whole grains with low-GI dried fruit
Vegetables and legumes	Pumpkin, parsnips, swedes, tapioca, most potatoes—steamed, boiled, mashed (new potatoes have the lowest GI value out of the common varieties tested so far, but are still medium GI)	Sweet potato, yams, taro, green peas, carrots, sweet corn, all legumes (dried, boiled, canned, vacuum-packed), non-starchy vegetables e.g. onions, tomatoes, lettuce, mushrooms, artichokes, asparagus, broccoli, cauliflower, ginger, garlic, cucumber, celery, capsicum (pepper), leeks, herbs
Fruit	Rockmelon, watermelon, sweetened dried cranberries, raisins, dried tenderized figs, lychees canned in syrup, dark cherries, breadfruit, pawpaw	Apples, pears, stone fruit (raw or canned in natural juice), berries, bananas (the less ripe, the lower the GI), kiwifruit, mango, custard apple, citrus fruit, grapes, some dried fruit e.g. prunes, dried apples, apricots, peaches, pears, sultanas
Dairy products and alternatives	Rice milk, sweetened condensed milk	Cows milk—plain or flavoured, all types, soy milk—plain or flavoured, all types, yoghurt, ice cream, custard pudding, fromage frais, diet jelly

Good sources of fibre

Food	Serve size	Approximate fibre content of serve (grams)
Processed wheat bran cereal (All-Bran)	¾ cup	15.1 g
Natural untoasted muesli (average)	⅔ cup	8.9 g
Bran flakes	1 cup	6.5 g
Oat bran, unprocessed	1 tbsp	1.8 g
Wheat bran, unprocessed	1 tbsp	2.2 g
Wholegrain bread, regular, supermarket variety	2 slices	3.3 g
Pumpernickel bread	1 slice	4.2 g
Brown rice, boiled or steamed	1 cup	2.7 g
Wholemeal (whole-wheat) pasta, boiled	1 cup	8.4 g
Barley, boiled	½ cup	3.3 g
Baked beans, tinned	¾ cup	9.9 g
Chickpeas, tinned, drained	½ cup	4.1 g
Kidney beans, tinned, drained	½ cup	6.2 g
Figs, dried	3 figs	8.1 g
Apricots, dried	8 halves	2.6 g
Strawberries, fresh	½ cup halves	1.8 g
Apple, raw, unpeeled	1 medium	3.3 g
Pear, green, raw, unpeeled	1 medium	3.7 g
Orange, raw, peeled	1 medium	2.6 g
Nectarine, raw, unpeeled	1 medium	3.6 g
Sauerkraut, tinned	½ cup	2.1 g
Broccoli, cooked	1 cup	4.2 g
Corn, cooked	1 medium cob	2.4 g
Green beans, cooked	½ cup	2.0 g
Spinach, cooked	½ cup chopped	4.6 g
Peas, green, cooked	½ cup	4.6 g
Brussels sprouts, cooked	4 sprouts	2.9 g
Potato, cooked whole, with skin	1 medium	2.8 g
Almonds, raw	⅓ cup	4.4 g
Pistachios, raw	⅓ cup	3.7 g
Peanuts, raw	⅓ cup	4.2 g
Sunflower seeds or pepitas (pumpkin seeds)	1 tbsp	1.4 g

Tips for increasing your fibre intake

- Choose wholegrain bread instead of white or wholemeal (whole-wheat).

- Choose brown rice and wholemeal (whole-wheat) pasta instead of white.

- Serve main meals with salads and plenty of vegetables.

- Eat whole fruit rather than drinking fruit juice.

- Have fruit-based desserts.

- Snack on dried fruit, fresh fruit, fresh vegetable sticks, nuts and seeds.

- Add boiled or tinned drained legumes to salads, soups, stews and curries.

- Choose a high-fibre breakfast cereal (natural muesli, bran-based cereals, psyllium-enriched flakes) and serve with fresh or dried fruit.

- Add some seeds or nuts to fruit salad, yoghurt, fruit crumbles and baking recipes.

- Make porridge from traditional wholegrain oats rather than quick-cooking or instant oats.

- Use wholemeal (whole-wheat) flour or stone-ground flour in baking recipes.

- Eat more vegetarian meals and stir-fries with lots of vegetables.

- Include lots of salad vegetables or tabouleh in your sandwiches and bread rolls.

- Explore your local health food shop to find high-fibre breakfast cereals, breads and snacks.

- Serve a variety of salads (bean salads, tabouleh) and different grainy breads at barbecues and picnics.

- Spray vegetables with olive oil and add them to the barbecue.

- When you serve rice, add some lentils or barley for extra fibre, nutrients and flavour. This will also lower the GI of the rice.

- If you want second helpings at dinner, make sure it's mostly vegetables.

- Add coarsely grated vegetables to cakes and muffins; and add more vegetables to pasta sauces, soups, stews and stir-fries.

- Make your own lunches for school or work. Try minestrone soup, salad or grainy bread rolls.

- Add vegetables to your breakfast by including them in omelettes or serving eggs with mushrooms, asparagus, tomatoes, spinach and wholegrain toast.

Comparison of daily fibre intake from low-fibre and high-fibre diets

Low fibre	(grams fibre)	High fibre	(grams fibre)
Breakfast			
Puffed rice cereal	0.7	Natural muesli	6.4
Reduced-fat milk	0.0	Reduced-fat milk	0.0
White sugar	0.0	Unpeeled nectarine	3.1
		1 tbsp sunflower seeds	1.2
Morning snack			
Apple juice	0.5	Water	0.0
Blueberry muffin	1.3	Whole apple, including skin	3.2
Lunch			
Ham and tomato sandwich (white bread)	2.3	Ham and salad sandwich (grainy bread)	4.5
Flavoured milk	0.0	Whole orange	2.6
Dinner			
White rice	1.0	Brown rice	2.9
Beef and vegetable stir-fry	1.5	Beef and vegetable stir-fry (with more vegetables)	2.5
Dessert			
Small serve tinned fruit	1.7	Fresh fruit salad	5.9
Ice cream	0.0	Ice cream	0.0
Total fibre intake	**9.0**		**32.3**

How to use this book

The recipes in this book have all been selected because they contain good amounts of fibre and meet other healthy eating guidelines. The nutrient content for an average serve is listed for each recipe. This is an estimate only, and can vary depending on the brand of ingredients used and due to variation in the nutrient content of natural produce. If the weight or amount of an ingredient is not specified, average or medium weights were used in the nutritional analysis. The nutritional analysis of recipes does not include any serving suggestions or garnishes, unless listed in specific quantities.

Disclaimer

This book provides general information about healthy eating based on valid information at the time of printing. It is not intended to replace any advice given to you by a qualified doctor or other mainstream health professional. If you have health problems and/or are taking prescription medication, it is particularly important that you consult with your doctor before making any changes to your dietary or exercise habits. Neither the author nor the publishers can be held responsible for claims arising from the inappropriate use or incorrect interpretation of any of the dietary advice described in this book.

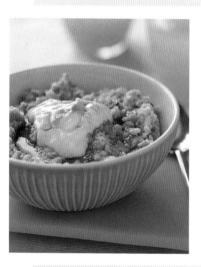

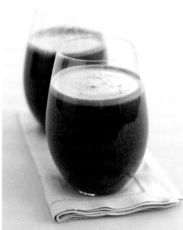

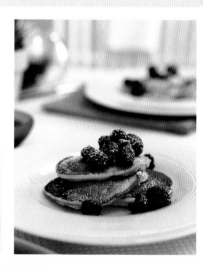

Breakfast

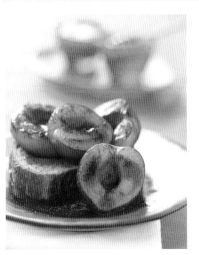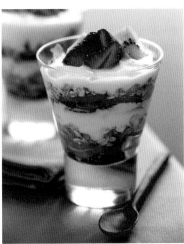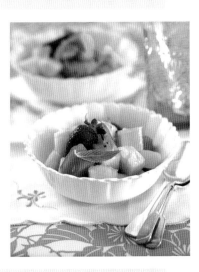

nutrition per serve   Energy 627 kJ (150 Cal) Fat 0.6 g Saturated fat 0 g
Protein 2.9 g Carbohydrate 30.1 g Fibre 5.2 g Cholesterol 0 mg Sodium 20 mg

Fruit salad with ginger lime syrup

½ small ripe pineapple, cut into
  3 cm (1¼ in) cubes

250 g (9 oz/1⅔ cups) strawberries,
  halved

500 g (1 lb 2 oz) peeled watermelon,
  cut into 3 cm (1¼ in) cubes

300 g (10½ oz) peeled rockmelon or
  any orange-fleshed melon, cut
  into 3 cm (1¼ in) cubes

½ papaya, cut into 3 cm (1¼ in)
  cubes

3 tbsp small mint leaves

45 g (1½ oz/¼ cup) soft brown sugar

125 ml (4 fl oz/½ cup) lime juice

2 cm (¾ in) piece fresh ginger,
  shredded

low-fat yoghurt, to serve

1 Put the fresh fruit and mint in a large bowl and gently
mix together.

2 Put the sugar, lime juice and 125 ml (4 fl oz/½ cup)
water in a small saucepan. Stir over low heat until the
sugar has dissolved. Add the ginger and bring to the
boil, then reduce the heat and simmer for 10 minutes,
or until the syrup has reduced a little.

3 Leave the syrup to cool, then pour over the fruit salad
and refrigerate until cold. Serve topped with yoghurt.

Prep time 15 minutes
Cooking time 15 minutes
Serves 4

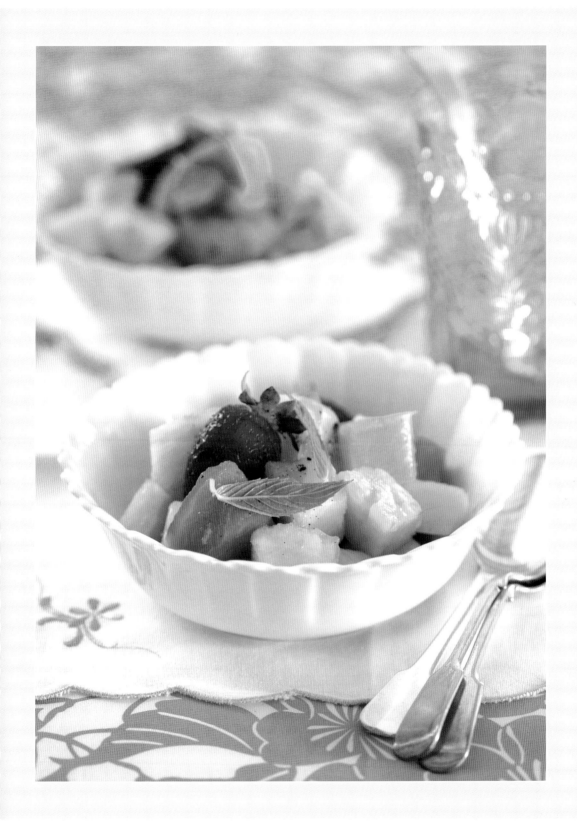

nutrition per serve
Energy 1761 kJ (421 Cal) Fat 11.4 g Saturated fat 1.4 g
Protein 10.8 g Carbohydrate 64 g Fibre 12.8 g Cholesterol 0 mg Sodium 57 mg

Full-of-fibre muesli

30 g (1 oz/⅓ cup) flaked almonds

200 g (7 oz/2 cups) wholegrain rolled
   (porridge) oats

60 g (2¼ oz/1 cup) processed
   bran cereal

35 g (1¼ oz/⅓ cup) wholegrain
   rolled barley

30 g (1 oz/¼ cup) pepitas
   (pumpkin seeds)

2 tbsp sunflower seeds

1 tbsp linseeds (flax seeds)

90 g (3¼ oz/¾ cup) sultanas
   (golden raisins)

185 g (6¼ oz/1 cup) chopped
   dried apricots

90 g (3¼ oz/½ cup) chopped
   dried pears

skim milk, to serve

low-fat yoghurt, to serve

Prep time 15 minutes

Cooking time 5 minutes

Serves 6

1 Preheat the oven to 160°C (315°F/Gas 2–3). Put the almonds on a baking tray in a single layer and toast in the oven for 5 minutes, or until golden. Remove and set aside.

2 Put the rolled oats, processed bran cereal, rolled barley, pepitas, sunflower seeds and linseeds in a bowl, then stir to combine. Add the sultanas, apricots and pears to the bowl, then stir in the toasted almonds.

3 Serve with skim milk and top with some yoghurt. Add some chopped fresh fruit for extra fibre, if desired. Store any remaining muesli in an airtight container for up to 2 weeks.

Multigrain porridge

400 g (14 oz/4 cups) wholegrain rolled (porridge) oats

100 g (3½ oz/1 cup) rice flakes

130 g (4½ oz/1 cup) barley flakes

130 g (4½ oz/1 cup) rye flakes

200 g (7 oz/1 cup) millet

2 tbsp sesame seeds, lightly toasted

2 tsp linseeds (flax seeds)

low-fat milk or plain yoghurt, to serve

soft brown sugar, to serve

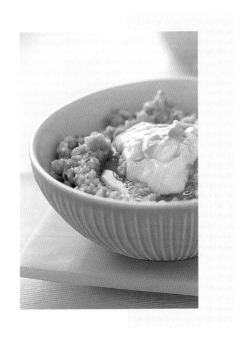

1   Put the rolled oats, rice flakes, barley flakes, rye flakes, millet, sesame seeds and linseeds in a large bowl and stir well. Store in a sealed container until ready to use.

2   To prepare the porridge for four people, put 250 g (9 oz/2 cups) of the dry mixture, a pinch of salt and 500 ml (17 fl oz/2 cups) water in a saucepan. Stir well, then set aside for 10 minutes (this creates a smoother, creamier porridge). Stir again and then add another 500 ml (17 fl oz/2 cups) water.

3   Bring to the boil over medium heat, stirring occasionally. Reduce the heat to low and simmer the porridge, stirring frequently, for 12–15 minutes, or until the mixture is soft and creamy and the grains are cooked. Serve with milk or yoghurt and brown sugar.

Prep time 10 minutes +
10 minutes soaking
Cooking time 20 minutes
Makes 16 serves

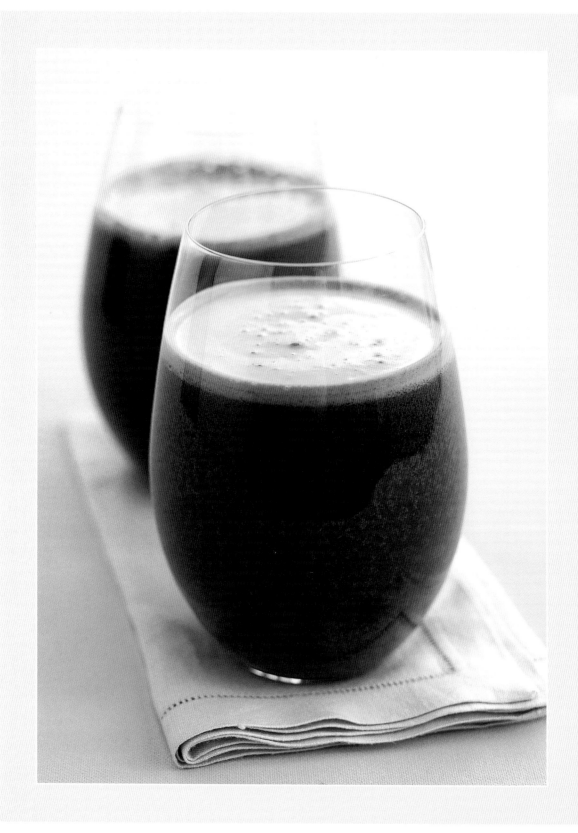

nutrition per serve Energy **879 kJ (210 Cal)** Fat **0.6 g** Saturated **fat 0 g**
Protein **4.4 g** Carbohydrate **40.1 g** Fibre **10 g** Cholesterol **0 mg** Sodium **30 mg**

Vegetable juice

1 beetroot (beet), scrubbed

10–12 carrots

2 green apples, stalks removed

2 large English spinach leaves

2 celery stalks

1 Wash the vegetables and cut them into pieces so they will fit into your juice extractor. Juice the beetroot, carrots, apples, spinach and celery in the juice extractor.

2 Return some of the pulp left in the extractor to the juice (the pulp contains lots of fibre). Stir well to combine and serve chilled.

Prep time 10 minutes

Cooking time Nil

Serves 2

nutrition per serve Energy **1825 kJ (436 Cal)** Fat **0.6 g** Saturated fat **0.1 g**
Protein **8.7 g** Carbohydrate **96.3 g** Fibre **7.9 g** Cholesterol **6 mg** Sodium **55 mg**

Orchard fruit compote

90 g (3¼ oz/¼ cup) honey

½ tsp ground ginger

1 cinnamon stick

3 whole cloves

pinch of ground nutmeg

750 ml (26 fl oz/3 cups) unsweetened
    apple juice

1 lemon

6 pitted prunes

3 dried peaches, halved

5 dates, halved and stones removed

10 dried apricots

1 lapsang souchong tea bag

2 golden delicious apples

2 beurre bosc pears

400 g (14 oz/1⅔ cups) low-fat
    vanilla yoghurt

Prep time 15 minutes +
30 minutes refrigeration
Cooking time 45 minutes
Serves 4

1 Put the honey, ginger, cinnamon stick, cloves, nutmeg and apple juice in a saucepan. Slice off a large piece of peel from the lemon and place in the pan. Squeeze the lemon to give 3 tablespoons juice, and add to the pan. Bring to the boil, stirring, then reduce the heat and simmer for 20 minutes.

2 Meanwhile, put the prunes, peaches, dates and apricots in a large heatproof bowl. Cover with boiling water, add the tea bag and leave to soak.

3 Peel and core the apples and pears, and cut into neat pieces about the same size as the dried fruits. Add to the syrup in the pan and simmer for 8–10 minutes, or until tender. Drain the dried fruit and discard the tea bag, then add the dried fruit to the pan and cook for a further 5 minutes.

4 Remove all the fruit from the pan with a slotted spoon, discard the lemon peel and place the fruit in a serving dish. Return the pan to the heat, bring to the boil, then reduce the heat and simmer for 6 minutes, or until the syrup has reduced by half. Pour the syrup over the fruit compote and refrigerate for 30 minutes. Serve with the yoghurt.

nutrition per serve (6) Energy **1278 kJ (305 Cal)** Fat **8.1 g** Saturated fat **0.8 g**
Protein **8.9 g** Carbohydrate **45.6 g** Fibre **7.1 g** Cholesterol **0 mg** Sodium **10 mg**

Dried fruit and nut quinoa

200 g (7 oz/1 cup) quinoa

500 ml (17 fl oz/2 cups) unsweetened apple juice

1 strip of orange peel

4 dried figs, chopped

4 dried peaches or dried pears, chopped

40 g (1½ oz/¼ cup) chopped raw almonds or hazelnuts

30 g (1 oz/¼ cup) pepitas (pumpkin seeds)

2 tsp grated orange zest

200 g (7 oz/1⅓ cups) strawberries, hulled and chopped

low-fat plain yoghurt, to serve

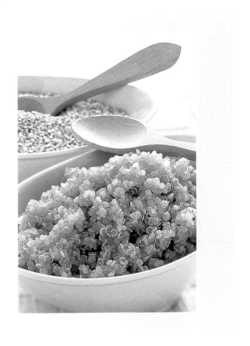

1 Put the quinoa in a sieve and rinse well under cold running water, then drain. Put the quinoa, apple juice and strip of orange peel in a saucepan.

2 Bring to the boil, then reduce the heat, cover and simmer for 10–15 minutes, or until all the liquid has been absorbed and the quinoa is translucent and the spiral germ ring is visible. Remove the orange peel. Cover the pan and set aside to allow the quinoa to firm up and cool a little.

3 Combine the dried fruit, nuts and pepitas. Add the orange zest and half the dried fruit mixture to the quinoa and stir well to combine. Spoon the mixture into four bowls and sprinkle with the remaining fruit mixture. Serve immediately, topped with the strawberries and yoghurt.

Prep time 15 minutes
Cooking time 15 minutes
Serves 4–6

nutrition per serve   Energy **1238 kJ (296 Cal)** Fat **4 g** Saturated fat **1 g**
Protein **11.8 g** Carbohydrate **48.8 g** Fibre **7.3 g** Cholesterol **5 mg** Sodium **105 mg**

Breakfast deluxe yoghurt

12 strawberries

4 kiwi fruit

**160 g (5½ oz/1½ cups) low-fat
natural muesli**

**400 g (14 oz/1⅔ cups) low-fat
plain yoghurt**

2 tbsp honey

Prep time 15 minutes

Cooking time Nil

Serves 4

1   Thinly slice the strawberries. Peel and thinly slice the kiwi fruit.

2   Place a few slices of strawberry in the bottom of each of four glasses. Top with a few slices of kiwi fruit, then top with some muesli and yoghurt. Repeat these layers again, reserving some of the fruit, and finishing with the yoghurt. Garnish with the reserved fruit and drizzle with the honey.

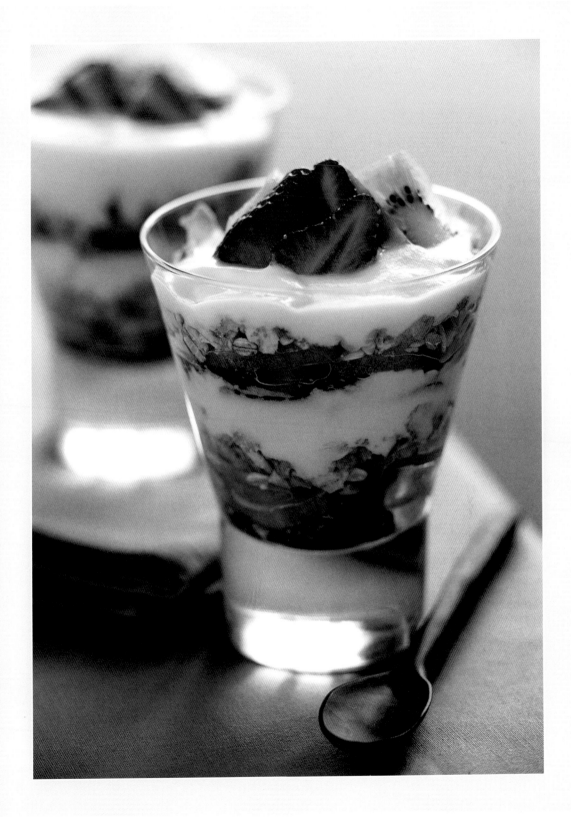

Savoury french toast

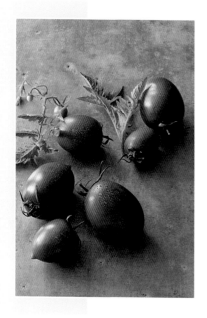

olive oil spray

4 vine-ripened tomatoes, halved

125 g (4½ oz/1 cup) grated low-fat cheddar cheese

1 small handful basil, plus extra, to garnish

8 slices soy and linseed bread

2 eggs

3 tbsp low-fat milk

25 g (1 oz) reduced-fat margarine

Prep time 15 minutes
Cooking time 20 minutes
Serves 4

1   Spray a non-stick frying pan with oil and heat over high heat. Add the tomatoes, cut side down, and fry for 1–2 minutes until tinged with brown. Remove and keep warm in a low oven. Wipe the pan clean.

2   Divide the cheese and basil among four slices of the bread, then top with the remaining bread slices. Press down well to form a tight sandwich.

3   Beat the eggs and milk together in a wide bowl and season well with salt and pepper. Add a quarter of the margarine to the pan and heat over medium heat.

4   Dip the sandwiches in the egg mixture until the bread is saturated but not soggy. Drain off the excess egg mixture and cook the sandwiches for 2 minutes on each side, or until crisp and golden. (You may be able to cook two sandwiches at once, depending on the size of your pan.) Repeat with the remaining margarine and sandwiches. Cut the sandwiches in half and serve with the tomatoes.

Bagels with baked beans

425 g (15 oz) tin baked beans

200 g (7 oz/4 cups) baby English spinach leaves

4 wholegrain or pumpernickel bagels, halved

250 g (9 oz/1 cup) low-fat cottage cheese

2 tomatoes, sliced, to serve

1 Put the baked beans in a small saucepan and cook over medium heat for 3 minutes, or until warmed through.

2 Place the washed spinach in a saucepan, cover and cook over medium heat for 2 minutes, or until wilted.

3 Toast the bagel halves and top with the cottage cheese and spinach. Spoon the baked beans over the top and season with freshly ground black pepper. Serve with the tomato slices on the side.

Prep time 10 minutes

Cooking time 10 minutes

Serves 4

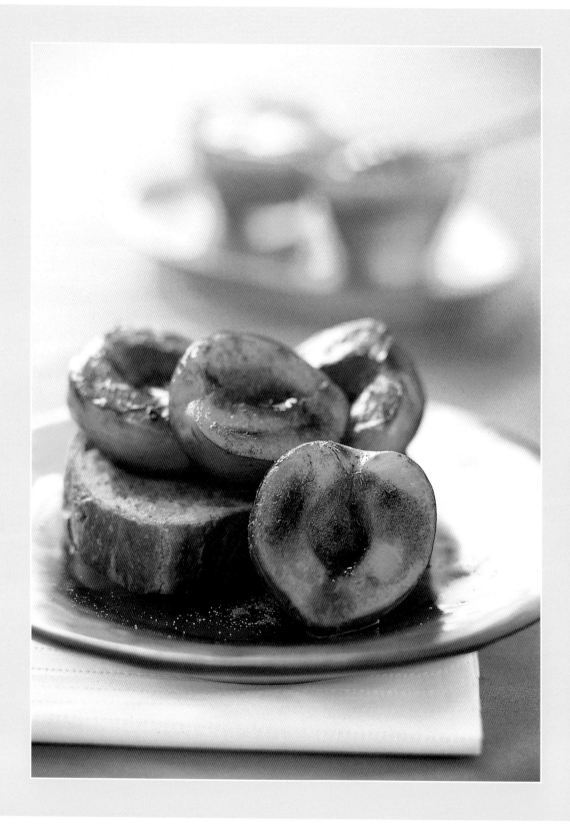

nutrition per serve   Energy **1737 kJ (415 Cal)** Fat **10.2 g** Saturated fat **4.5 g**
Protein **11.7 g** Carbohydrate **65.2 g** Fibre **6.6 g** Cholesterol **42 mg** Sodium **139 mg**

Stone fruits with cinnamon toast

1 tbsp reduced-fat margarine

½ tsp ground cinnamon

4 thick slices good-quality brioche

4 ripe plums, halved and stones removed

4 ripe nectarines, halved and stones removed

200 g (7 oz) low-fat vanilla fromage frais

2 tbsp warmed blossom honey

Prep time 10 minutes

Cooking time 10 minutes

Serves 4

1 Put the margarine and half the cinnamon in a bowl and mix until well combined. Place the slices of brioche under a preheated grill (broiler) and grill (broil) on one side until golden. Spread the untoasted side of the brioche slices using half the cinnamon margarine, then grill until golden. Keep the toast warm in the oven.

2 Brush the cut side of the plums and nectarines with the remaining margarine and cook under the grill, cut side up, or in a chargrill pan, cut side down, until the fruit is tinged brown at the edges.

3 To serve, place two plum halves and two nectarine halves on each toasted slice of brioche. Dollop a little fromage frais on top, dust with the remaining cinnamon and drizzle with the warmed honey.

nutrition per serve   Energy 2165 kJ (517 Cal) Fat 25.6 g Saturated fat 6.2 g
Protein 32 g Carbohydrate 35.3 g Fibre 9.1 g Cholesterol 563 mg Sodium 535 mg

Scrambled eggs with mushrooms

2 vine-ripened tomatoes, halved

4 field mushrooms

canola or olive oil spray

2 tsp thyme, plus extra, to garnish

6 eggs

1 tbsp reduced-fat milk

30 g (1 oz) reduced-fat canola or
   olive oil margarine

4 slices wholegrain bread, toasted

50 g (1¾ oz/1 cup) baby English
   spinach leaves

Prep time 10 minutes

Cooking time 10 minutes

Serves 2

1 Put the tomatoes, cut side up, and the mushrooms on a grill (broiler) tray. Spray with oil and scatter with the thyme leaves. Place the tray under a preheated grill and cook for 3–5 minutes, or until warmed.

2 Meanwhile, break the eggs into a bowl, add the milk and season well with salt and freshly ground black pepper. Whisk gently with a fork until well combined.

3 Melt half the margarine in a small non-stick saucepan or frying pan over low heat. Add the eggs, then stir constantly with a wooden spoon. Do not turn up the heat—scrambling needs to be done slowly and gently. When most of the egg has set, add the remaining margarine and remove the pan from the heat. There will be enough heat left in the pan to finish cooking the eggs and melt the margarine.

4 Serve the eggs immediately on toast. Arrange the tomatoes, mushrooms and spinach leaves on the side. Garnish the eggs with extra thyme.

Mixed fruit frappe

10 dried apricot halves

**200 g (7 oz) fresh or frozen
raspberries**

1 banana, roughly chopped

1 mango, roughly chopped

500 ml (17 fl oz/2 cups) orange juice

1 tbsp mint leaves

6 ice cubes

1 Put the dried apricots in a heatproof bowl. Cover with 3 tablespoons boiling water and leave to soak for 10 minutes, or until plump. Drain and roughly chop.

2 Blend the chopped apricots, raspberries, banana, mango, orange juice, mint and ice in a blender until thick and smooth. Do not overblend the mixture—you want to leave some small chunks of fruit. Serve immediately.

Prep time 5 minutes +
10 minutes soaking

Cooking time Nil

Serves 4

Pancakes with maple raspberries

60 g (2¼ oz/½ cup) plain
   (all-purpose) flour

75 g (2½ oz/½ cup) wholemeal
   (whole-wheat) flour

50 g (1¾ oz/½ cup) soy flour

1 tbsp baking powder

2 tbsp sugar

65 g (2¼ oz) silken tofu

420 ml (14½ fl oz/1⅔ cups) low-fat
   soy milk

1 tsp natural vanilla extract

20 g (¾ oz) reduced-fat soy spread or
   margarine, melted

500 g (1 lb 2 oz/4 cups) raspberries

125 ml (4 fl oz/½ cup) pure maple
   syrup

icing (confectioners') sugar,
   for dusting

Prep time 10 minutes +
15 minutes standing

Cooking time 20 minutes

Serves 4–6

1 Sift the flours, baking powder and ½ teaspoon salt into a large bowl (return the husks to the bowl), then stir in the sugar. Place the tofu, soy milk and vanilla in a food processor and combine until the mixture is smooth. Add to the dry ingredients and mix together well. Cover with plastic wrap and leave for 15 minutes.

2 Brush a frying pan with some of the melted spread and heat over medium heat. Cooking two pancakes at a time, drop 2 tablespoons of batter per pancake into the pan, spreading the mixture out a little with the back of the spoon. Cook for 1–2 minutes, or until bubbles form on the surface. Flip the pancake over and cook the other side for 1 minute, or until golden. Keep warm and repeat with the remaining batter to make 12 pancakes in total.

3 Put the raspberries and maple syrup in a saucepan and stir to combine. Gently cook for 1–2 minutes, or until the berries are warm and well coated in the syrup. Place two or three pancakes on each plate, top with the maple raspberries and dust with icing sugar.

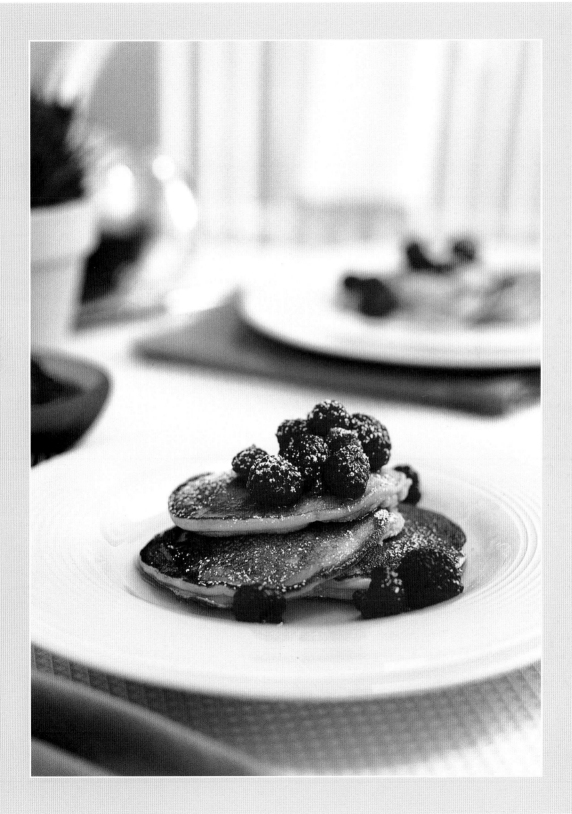

nutrition per serve   Energy **1298 kJ (310 Cal)** Fat **11.8 g** Saturated fat **3 g**
Protein **28.3 g** Carbohydrate **20.6 g** Fibre **4 g** Cholesterol **293 mg** Sodium **652 mg**

Smoked salmon omelette

175 g (6 oz/1 bunch) asparagus,
   ends trimmed, cut into 5 cm
   (2 in) lengths

3 egg whites

3 whole eggs

1 tbsp low-fat ricotta cheese

1 tbsp chopped dill

olive oil spray

50 g (1¾ oz/1 cup) baby English
   spinach leaves

50 g (1¾ oz) smoked salmon,
   thinly sliced

lemon wedges, to garnish

2 slices wholegrain bread, toasted

Prep time 10 minutes
Cooking time 10 minutes
Serves 2

1 Bring a saucepan of water to the boil. Then add the asparagus and cook for 30 seconds, then remove and refresh in cold water and drain.

2 Whisk the egg whites in a bowl until foaming. In a separate bowl, whisk together the whole eggs and ricotta cheese, then whisk in the egg whites until well combined. Stir in the dill and season with freshly ground black pepper.

3 Spray a 24 cm (9½ in) non-stick frying pan with oil and heat over low heat. Pour in half the egg mixture and arrange half the asparagus pieces evenly over the top. Scatter half the spinach over the top. Cook over medium heat until the egg is just set and the spinach has started to wilt slightly. Carefully flip one half of the omelette onto the other, then transfer to a serving plate and keep warm. Repeat with the remaining egg, asparagus and spinach to make a second omelette.

4 Top the omelettes with smoked salmon and garnish with wedges of lemon. Serve with wholegrain toast.

nutrition per serve Energy **1290 kJ (308 Cal)** Fat **1 g** Saturated fat **0.3 g**
Protein **15.5 g** Carbohydrate **57 g** Fibre **4.6 g** Cholesterol **10 mg** Sodium **110 mg**

Peach and banana smoothie

375 ml (13 fl oz/1½ cups) skim milk

150 g (5½ oz/⅔ cup) low-fat vanilla yoghurt

2 very ripe bananas, chopped

1 large yellow peach, chopped

2 tbsp wheat germ

1 tbsp pure maple syrup

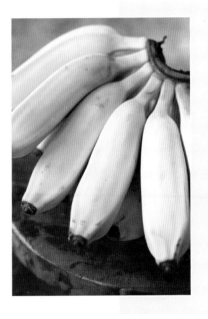

1 Blend the milk, yoghurt, bananas, peach, wheat germ and maple syrup in a blender until combined. Do not overblend the mixture—you want to leave some small chunks of fruit. Serve immediately.

Prep time 5 minutes
Cooking time Nil
Serves 2

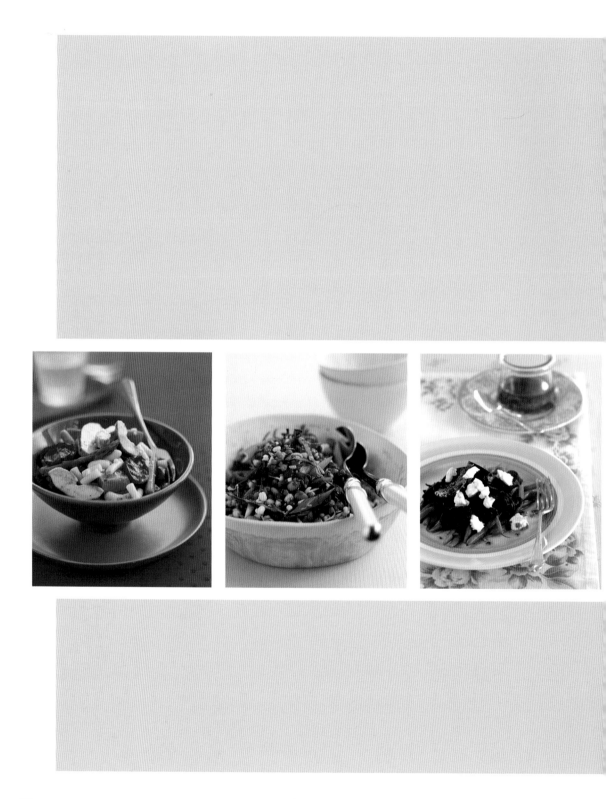

Salads and
light meals

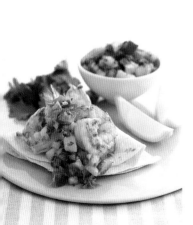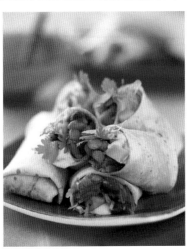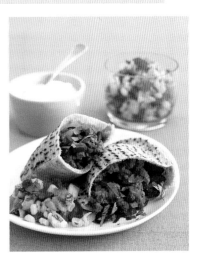

nutrition per serve Energy **424 kJ (101 Cal)** Fat **3.4 g** Saturated fat **0.5 g**
Protein **5.3 g** Carbohydrate **9.4 g** Fibre **6.2 g** Cholesterol **0 mg** Sodium **113 mg**

Sprout and cabbage salad

½ small red cabbage (600 g/1 lb 5 oz),
  core removed, finely shredded

420 g (15 oz) tin four bean mix,
  drained and rinsed

200 g (7 oz/2¼ cups) mung bean
  sprouts

4 large spring onions (scallions),
  sliced

Dressing

1 tbsp olive oil

2 tsp lemon juice

1 large garlic clove, crushed

Prep time 15 minutes
Cooking time Nil
Serves 6

1 Put the shredded cabbage, four bean mix, bean sprouts and spring onions in a large serving bowl. Mix together gently.

2 To make the dressing, whisk the olive oil and lemon juice together in a small bowl. Stir in the garlic and season with salt (if desired) and freshly ground black pepper. Pour the dressing over the salad and toss to combine.

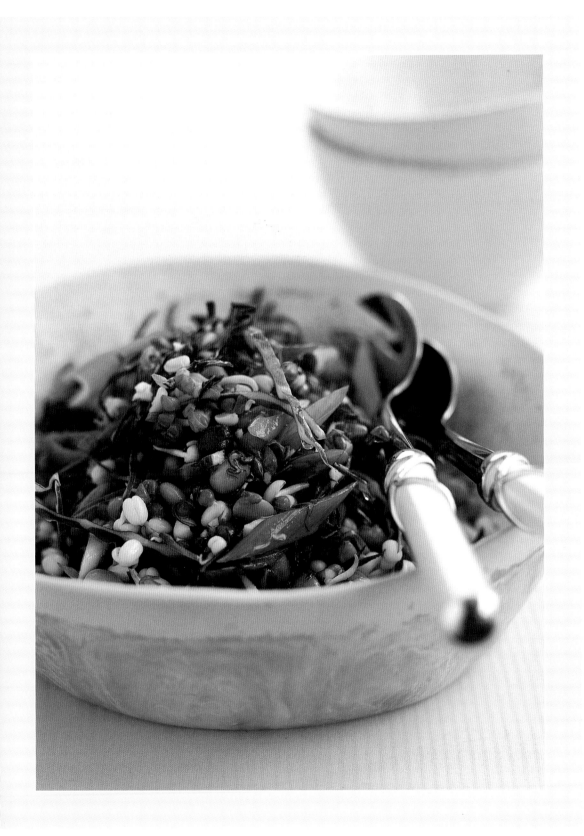

nutrition per serve Energy **1337 kJ (318 Cal)** Fat **10 g** Saturated fat **4 g**
Protein **29.8 g** Carbohydrate **23.4 g** Fibre **5.1 g** Cholesterol **59 mg** Sodium **648 mg**

Watercress and salmon salad

150 g (5½ oz) sugar snap peas

500 g (1 lb 2 oz) kipfler (fingerling) potatoes, scrubbed

300 g (10½ oz) watercress, washed and sprigs removed

2 Lebanese (short) cucumbers, halved lengthways, sliced on the diagonal

400 g (14 oz) smoked salmon, cut into 4 cm (1½ in) pieces

3 tbsp horseradish cream

2 garlic cloves, crushed

4 tbsp light sour cream

1 tsp grated lemon zest

3 tsp lemon juice

2 tsp chopped dill

1 Bring a large saucepan of water to the boil. Add the snap peas and blanch them until they are bright green. Remove with a slotted spoon, refresh under cold water and set aside.

2 Return the water to the boil and cook the potatoes for 8–10 minutes, or until tender, then drain well. Cut into 1.5 cm (⅝ in) slices on the diagonal. Cool.

3 Put the sugar snap peas, potatoes, watercress, cucumbers and smoked salmon in a large bowl. Combine the horseradish, garlic, sour cream, lemon zest, lemon juice and dill in a small bowl. Spoon the dressing over the salad and toss until well combined. Season with salt (if desired) and freshly ground black pepper. Serve immediately with crusty wholegrain bread.

Prep time 15 minutes

Cooking time 10 minutes

Serves 4

nutrition per serve (6)   Energy **848 kJ (202 Cal)** Fat **4.4 g** Saturated fat **1.6 g**
Protein **24.9 g** Carbohydrate **16.6 g** Fibre **7.1 g** Cholesterol **24 mg** Sodium **398 mg**

Tuna and cannellini bean salad

400 g (14 oz) tuna steaks

cracked black pepper

1 small red onion, thinly sliced

1 tomato, seeded and chopped

1 small red capsicum (pepper), thinly sliced

2 x 400 g (14 oz) tins cannellini beans, drained and rinsed

2 garlic cloves, crushed

1 tsp chopped thyme

4 tbsp finely chopped flat-leaf (Italian) parsley

4 tbsp fat-free French dressing

100 g (3½ oz) rocket (arugula) leaves

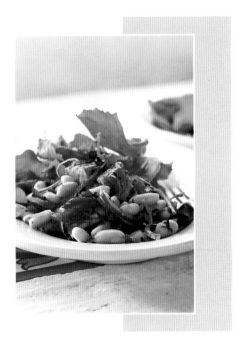

1 Put the tuna steaks on a plate, sprinkle with cracked black pepper on both sides, cover with plastic wrap and refrigerate until needed.

2 Combine the onion, tomato, capsicum and cannellini beans in a large bowl. Add the garlic, thyme and 3 tablespoons of the parsley and toss to combine.

3 Lightly oil a barbecue chargrill plate or hotplate and heat to high. Add the tuna and cook for 1 minute on each side. The tuna should still be pink in the middle. Cut the tuna into small cubes and combine with the salad. Pour over the dressing and toss to coat.

4 Arrange the rocket on a platter. Top with the tuna and bean salad, season with salt and freshly ground black pepper and sprinkle with the remaining parsley.

Prep time 25 minutes
Cooking time 2 minutes
Serves 4–6

Thai beef salad

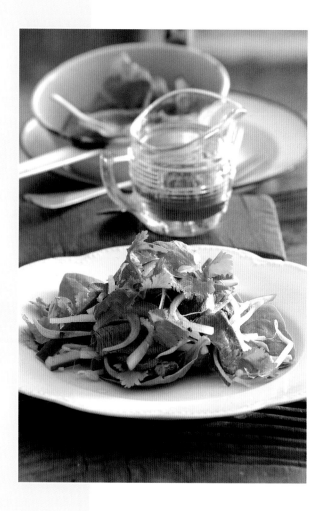

2 tbsp dried shrimp

200 g (7 oz) mixed lettuce leaves

2 tsp sesame oil

500 g (1 lb 2 oz) rump steak, trimmed

90 g (3¼ oz/1 cup) bean sprouts

1 small red onion, thinly sliced

1 red capsicum (pepper), cut into thin strips

1 Lebanese (short) cucumber, cut into thin strips

200 g (7 oz) daikon radish, peeled and cut into thin strips

250 g (9 oz) cherry tomatoes, halved

1 small handful mint

1 handful coriander (cilantro) leaves

1 handful Thai basil

2 garlic cloves, finely chopped

2 tbsp chopped toasted peanuts

nutrition per serve

Energy **1238 kJ (296 Cal)** Fat **12.3 g** Saturated fat **3.4 g**
Protein **33.8 g** Carbohydrate **9.2 g** Fibre **5.5 g** Cholesterol **81 mg** Sodium **1710 mg**

Dressing

3 tbsp lime juice

3 tbsp fish sauce

1 tbsp finely chopped lemon grass

1 red chilli, seeded and chopped

1 long green chilli, seeded and chopped

1 tsp sugar

Prep time 25 minutes +
15 minutes soaking
Cooking time 4 minutes
Serves 4

1 Soak the dried shrimp in hot water for 15 minutes, then drain well and finely chop. Wash the lettuce leaves and drain well.

2 Heat the oil in a frying pan over high heat, add the steak and cook until medium–rare, for about 1½–2 minutes on each side. Remove from the pan and leave to cool slightly. Slice the steak thinly.

3 To make the dressing, combine the lime juice, fish sauce, lemon grass, chillies and sugar in a small bowl. Whisk until the ingredients are combined and the sugar has dissolved.

4 Put the shrimp, the sliced beef, the bean sprouts, onion, capsicum, cucumber, radish, tomatoes, herbs and garlic in a large bowl and then toss to combine. Place the salad leaves on a serving plate, top with the beef and vegetables and drizzle with the dressing, using enough of the dressing to moisten the salad. Sprinkle with the chopped peanuts.

nutrition per serve   Energy **954 kJ (228 Cal)** Fat **13.4 g** Saturated fat **3.9 g**
Protein **7.8 g** Carbohydrate **15.9 g** Fibre **7.1 g** Cholesterol **10 mg** Sodium **500 mg**

Beetroot and goat's cheese salad

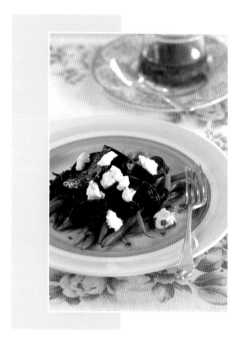

1 kg (2 lb 4 oz) beetroot (beets), with leaves (4 bulbs)

200 g (7 oz) green beans, trimmed

1 tbsp red wine vinegar

2 tbsp extra virgin olive oil

1 garlic clove, crushed

1 tbsp capers in brine, rinsed and roughly chopped

100 g (3½ oz) goat's cheese

Prep time 15 minutes

Cooking time 40 minutes

Serves 4

1 Trim the leaves from the beetroot, leaving about 3 cm (1¼ in) of stalk attached to the bulb. Scrub bulbs and wash leaves. Bring a large saucepan of water to the boil, add beetroot, then reduce the heat and simmer, covered, for 30 minutes, or until tender when pierced with a knife. (The cooking time may vary depending on the size of the bulbs.) Drain and cool. Peel the skins off the beetroot and cut the bulbs into wedges.

2 Meanwhile, bring a saucepan of water to the boil, add beans and cook for 3 minutes. Remove with tongs and place in a bowl of cold water. Drain well. Add beetroot leaves to boiled water and cook for 3–5 minutes over medium heat until the leaves and stems are tender. Drain, transfer to a bowl of cold water, then drain well.

3 To make the dressing, put vinegar, oil, garlic, capers and ½ teaspoon freshly ground black pepper into a screw-top jar and shake well. Taste for seasoning. To serve, divide beans, beetroot wedges and leaves among four plates. Crumble goat's cheese over the top and drizzle with the dressing.

nutrition per serve (10)   Energy 554 kJ (132 Cal) Fat 1.1 g Saturated fat 0.1 g
Protein 6.8 g Carbohydrate 20.4 g Fibre 6.7 g Cholesterol 0 mg Sodium 510 mg

Three bean salad

250 g (9 oz) green beans, trimmed

400 g (14 oz) tin chickpeas, drained and rinsed

400 g (14 oz) tin red kidney beans, drained and rinsed

400 g (14 oz) tin cannellini beans, drained and rinsed

310 g (11 oz) tin corn kernels, drained and rinsed

3 spring onions (scallions), sliced

1 red capsicum (pepper), chopped

3 celery stalks, chopped

4–6 gherkins (pickles), chopped

3 tbsp chopped mint

3 tbsp chopped flat-leaf (Italian) parsley

Mustard vinaigrette

125 ml (4 fl oz/½ cup) fat-free French dressing

1 tbsp dijon mustard

1 garlic clove, crushed

1 Cut the green beans into short lengths. Bring a small saucepan of water to the boil, add the beans and cook for 2 minutes. Drain and rinse under cold water, then leave in iced water until cold. Drain.

2 Put the green beans, chickpeas, kidney beans, cannellini beans, corn, spring onions, capsicum, celery, gherkin, mint and parsley in a large bowl. Season with salt (if desired) and freshly ground black pepper and mix together.

3 To make the vinaigrette, put the dressing, mustard and garlic in a small bowl and whisk until well blended. Drizzle the vinaigrette over the salad and toss gently.

Prep time 15 minutes
Cooking time 2 minutes
Serves 8–10

nutrition per serve Energy **1857 kJ (444 Cal)** Fat **2.8 g** Saturated fat **0.7 g**
Protein **29.3 g** Carbohydrate **70.4 g** Fibre **8.8 g** Cholesterol **47 mg** Sodium **283 mg**

Chicken, bean and pasta salad

**750 g (1 lb 10 oz) orange sweet
    potato, peeled and cut into
    2 cm (¾ in) cubes**

250 g (9 oz) cherry tomatoes, halved

olive oil spray

**2 x 200 g (7 oz) boneless, skinless
    chicken breasts**

**350 g (12 oz/2 bunches) asparagus,
    trimmed and cut into thirds**

375 g (13 oz) macaroni

**400 g (14 oz) tin cannellini beans,
    drained and rinsed**

**3 handfuls baby rocket (arugula)
    leaves**

3 tbsp fat-free French dressing

Prep time 15 minutes
Cooking time 1 hour
Serves 6

1 Preheat the oven to 200°C (400°F/Gas 6). Put the sweet potato in one end of a large non-stick roasting tin and the tomatoes in the other end, cut side down. Lightly spray with oil and bake for 45 minutes, turning halfway through cooking time. Remove the tomatoes after 30 minutes.

2 Meanwhile, lightly spray a chargrill pan or barbecue chargrill plate with oil and heat to high. Cook chicken for 5 minutes on each side, or until cooked through.

3 Bring a large saucepan of water to the boil. Add the asparagus and cook for 1 minute, then remove with a slotted spoon and place into iced water. Drain. Return the water to the boil and cook the macaroni for 10 minutes, or until tender. Drain and keep warm.

4 Slice the chicken into 1 cm (½ in) thick strips and place in a large bowl with the roasted sweet potato and tomatoes, asparagus, pasta, beans and rocket and toss until combined. Add the dressing to the salad and toss until well combined. Season with salt (if desired) and freshly ground black pepper and serve immediately.

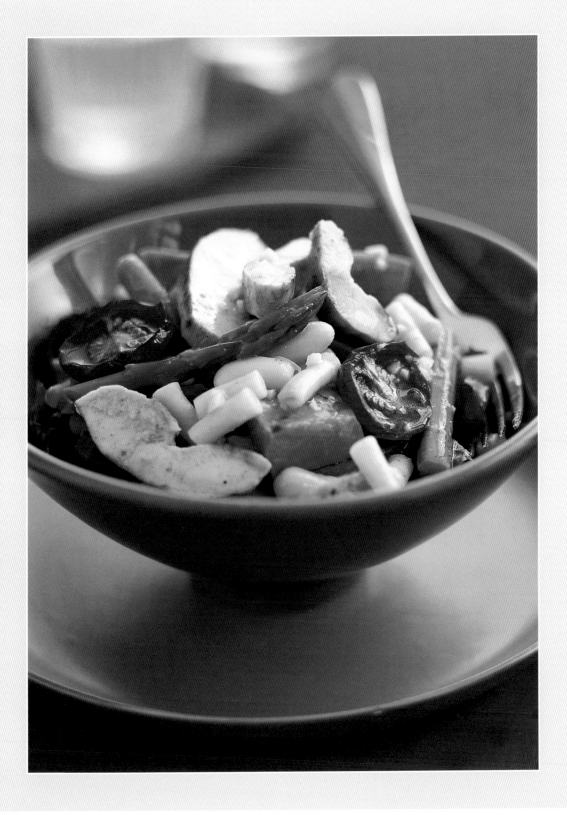

Lamb and pasta salad

100 g (3½ oz) sun-dried tomatoes
(not packed in oil)

500 g (1 lb 2 oz) broad (fava) beans,
to yield about 175 g (6 oz)
podded beans

375 g (13 oz) wholemeal
(whole-wheat) pasta

1 tablespoon olive oil

1 red onion, chopped

2 garlic cloves, lightly crushed

3 tomatoes, chopped

350 g (12 oz) lean lamb loin

100 g (3½ oz/2 cups) baby English
spinach leaves

1 tbsp lemon juice

40 g (1½ oz/¼ cup) pine nuts,
lightly toasted

Prep time 15 minutes +
10 minutes soaking
Cooking time 25 minutes
Serves 6

1   Pour boiling water over the sun-dried tomatoes and set
aside to soften for 10 minutes, then drain and chop.
Peel the podded broad beans and blanch them in a
saucepan of boiling water for 2 minutes. Drain and
refresh in cold water.

2   Bring a large saucepan of water to the boil, add the
pasta and cook for 12 minutes, or until al dente. Drain
and reserve 125 ml (4 fl oz/½ cup) of pasta water.

3   While the pasta is cooking, heat the oil in a large frying
pan, add the onion and cook for 2–3 minutes, then add
the garlic and cook for a further 2 minutes. Remove to a
large bowl with a slotted spoon and stir in the chopped
fresh tomatoes. Reheat the pan and, when hot, add the
lamb. Brown well on both sides, then cook for a further
2–3 minutes on each side until just cooked. The flesh
will still be slightly pink in the centre. Cover and set
aside for 5 minutes, then thinly slice the lamb on the
diagonal.

4   Add the sun-dried tomatoes, broad beans and lamb to
the onion and tomato mixture and gently combine.
Toss through the hot pasta, adding the spinach,
reserved water and the lemon juice. Scatter over the
pine nuts and toss to combine. Divide among serving
plates, season with freshly ground black pepper and
serve immediately.

nutrition per serve (6)

Energy **722 kJ (172 Cal)** Fat **11.8 g** Saturated fat **1.6 g**
Protein **4.4 g** Carbohydrate **10.6 g** Fibre **4.8 g** Cholesterol **0 mg** Sodium **84 mg**

Pear and bean salad

2 pears, unpeeled, cored and chopped

45 g (1½ oz/½ cup) bean sprouts

125 g (4½ oz/1 cup) sliced, cooked green beans

4 spring onions (scallions), chopped

125 g (4½ oz) tin red kidney beans, drained and rinsed

100 g (3½ oz/½ cup) drained and rinsed tinned
    soya beans, or use frozen

1 tbsp poppy seeds

Dressing

3 tbsp olive oil

1 tsp white vinegar

½ tsp sugar

1 garlic clove, crushed

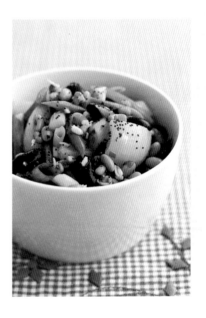

1 Combine the pears, bean sprouts, green beans, spring
onions, kidney beans and soya beans in a large bowl.
Mix together gently.

2 To make the dressing, combine the oil, vinegar, sugar,
garlic and 3 tablespoons water. Taste for seasoning,
then pour over the vegetables. Chill the salad for an
hour before serving. Sprinkle with the poppy seeds
just before you are ready to serve.

Prep time 20 minutes +
1 hour refrigeration
Cooking time Nil
Serves 4–6

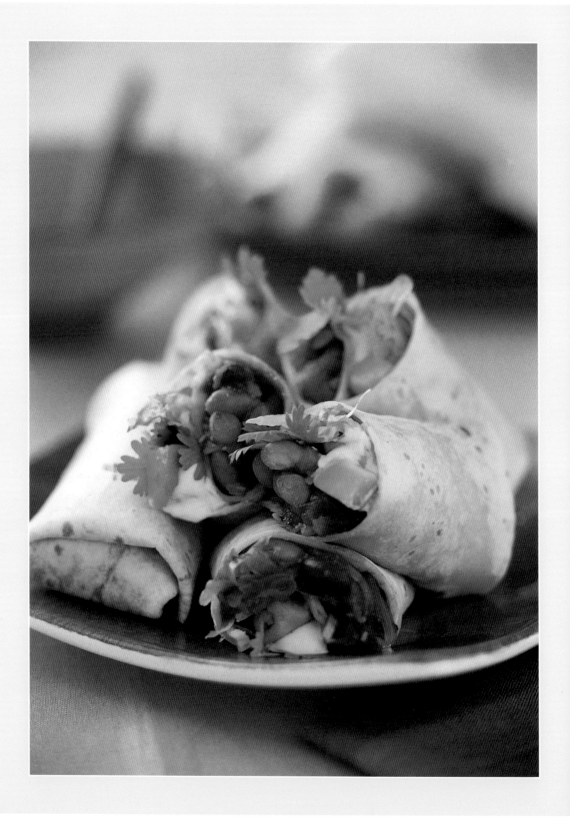

nutrition per enchilada
Energy **993 kJ (237 Cal)** Fat **11.1 g** Saturated fat **2.8 g** Protein **8.5 g** Carbohydrate **22.8 g** Fibre **6.5 g** Cholesterol **10 mg** Sodium **301 mg**

Bean enchiladas

1 tbsp light olive oil

1 onion, thinly sliced

3 garlic cloves, crushed

1 bird's eye chilli, finely chopped

2 tsp ground cumin

125 ml (4 fl oz/½ cup) vegetable stock

3 tomatoes, peeled, seeded and chopped

1 tbsp tomato paste (concentrated purée)

2 x 420 g (15 oz) tins three bean mix, drained and rinsed

2 tbsp chopped coriander (cilantro) leaves

8 flour tortillas

1 small avocado, chopped

125 g (4½ oz/½ cup) light sour cream

1 handful coriander (cilantro) sprigs

115 g (4 oz/2 cups) shredded lettuce

1 Heat the olive oil in a deep frying pan over medium heat. Add the onion and cook for 3–4 minutes, or until just soft. Add the garlic and chilli and cook for a further 30 seconds. Add the cumin, stock, tomatoes and tomato paste and cook for 6–8 minutes, or until the mixture is quite thick and pulpy. Season with salt (if desired) and freshly ground black pepper.

2 Preheat the oven to 170°C (325°F/Gas 3). Add the bean mix to the sauce and cook for 5 minutes to heat through, then add the chopped coriander.

3 Meanwhile, wrap the tortillas in foil and warm in the oven for 3–4 minutes.

4 Place a warm tortilla on a plate and spread with some of the bean mixture. Top with some avocado, sour cream, coriander sprigs and lettuce. Roll the enchiladas up, tucking in the ends. Cut each one in half to serve.

Prep time 20 minutes

Cooking time 20 minutes

Makes 8

nutrition per serve Energy **1347 kJ (322 Cal)** Fat **4.7 g** Saturated fat **1.4 g**
Protein **15.8 g** Carbohydrate **49.2 g** Fibre **9.4 g** Cholesterol **15 mg** Sodium **307 mg**

Pizzette

300 g (10½ oz/2 cups) wholemeal (whole-wheat) flour

2 tsp dry yeast

½ tsp sugar

2 tbsp plain yoghurt

Topping

2 tbsp tomato paste (concentrated purée)

1 garlic clove, crushed

1 tsp dried oregano

80 g (2¾ oz) lean shaved ham, sliced into strips

2 tbsp grated light mozzarella cheese

20 g (¾ oz) baby rocket (arugula) leaves, torn

extra virgin olive oil, to drizzle

Prep time 10 minutes +
20–30 minutes standing

Cooking time 12–15 minutes

Serves 4

1 Sift the flour into a bowl, then return the husks to the bowl. Add the yeast, sugar and ½ teaspoon salt. Make a well in the centre, add 125 ml (4 fl oz/½ cup) water and the yoghurt and mix to form a dough.

2 Knead on a lightly floured surface for 5 minutes, or until smooth and elastic. Place the dough in a lightly oiled bowl, cover with a tea towel (dish towel) and rest in a warm place for 20–30 minutes, or until doubled in size. Preheat the oven to 200ºC (400°F/Gas 6).

3 Punch the dough down and knead for 30 seconds, then divide into four portions. Roll each portion into a 15 cm (6 in) round and place on a baking tray.

4 To make the topping, combine the tomato paste, garlic, oregano and 1 tablespoon water. Spread the paste over each base, then top each with some shaved ham and mozzarella. Bake for 12–15 minutes, or until crisp and golden on the edges. Just before serving, top with the torn rocket and drizzle with extra virgin olive oil. Serve with a vinegar-dressed mixed leaf salad, if desired.

nutrition per serve Energy 1475 kJ (352 Cal) Fat 6.8 g Saturated fat 0.8 g
Protein 11.5 g Carbohydrate 57.1 g Fibre 9 g Cholesterol 0 mg Sodium 1260 mg

Sweet potato and lentil rissoles

400 g (14 oz) tin brown lentils,
    drained and rinsed

1 small onion, finely chopped

1 small green capsicum (pepper),
    finely chopped

1 carrot, grated

2 tbsp chopped flat-leaf (Italian)
    parsley

425 g (15 oz/1⅓ cups) cooked and
    mashed sweet potato

160 g (5½ oz/2 cups) fresh
    wholegrain breadcrumbs
    (2–3 slices bread)

1 tsp ground cumin

dry wholegrain breadcrumbs,
    for coating

olive oil spray

Sauce

185 ml (6 fl oz/¾ cup) tomato sauce
    (ketchup)

1–2 tsp curry powder

2 tsp lemon juice

1 Combine the lentils, onion, capsicum, carrot and parsley in a large bowl. Use clean hands to combine and then mix in the mashed sweet potato, breadcrumbs and cumin. Season well with salt (if desired) and freshly ground black pepper. Divide the mixture into eight even-sized patties and refrigerate for at least 30 minutes to firm up and develop flavour.

2 Preheat the oven to 200°C (400°F/Gas 6). Line a baking tray with baking paper.

3 Coat the rissoles in the dry breadcrumbs and spray the rissoles with the oil. Place on the prepared tray and bake, turning once or twice, for 35 minutes, or until crisp and golden.

4 Meanwhile, combine the sauce ingredients in a small saucepan and bring to the boil. Set aside. Serve rissoles hot or cold with the tomato sauce and a mixed salad.

Prep time 20 minutes +
30 minutes refrigeration
Cooking time 40 minutes
Serves 4

nutrition per serve Energy **1313 kJ (314 Cal)** Fat **9.5 g** Saturated fat **2.9 g**
Protein **14.4 g** Carbohydrate **39.6 g** Fibre **5.9 g** Cholesterol **102 mg** Sodium **113 mg**

Roast vegetable quiche

1 large potato, unpeeled

400 g (14 oz) peeled pumpkin
  (winter squash)

200 g (7 oz) orange sweet potato,
  unpeeled

2 large parsnips, unpeeled

1 red capsicum (pepper)

2 onions, cut into wedges

6 garlic cloves, halved

2 tsp olive oil

90 g (3¼ oz/¾ cup) plain
  (all-purpose) flour

75 g (2½ oz/½ cup) wholemeal
  (whole-wheat) flour

40 g (1½ oz) reduced-fat margarine

45 g (1½ oz) ricotta cheese

250 ml (9 fl oz/1 cup) skim milk

3 eggs, lightly beaten

30 g (1 oz/¼ cup) grated reduced-fat
  cheddar cheese

2 tbsp chopped basil

Prep time 45 minutes +
25 minutes refrigeration
Cooking time 2½ hours
Serves 6

1 Preheat the oven to 180°C (350°F/Gas 4). Lightly grease a 3.5 cm (1¼ in) deep, 23 cm (9 in) loose-based flan tin.

2 Cut the potato, pumpkin, sweet potato, parsnips and capsicum into bite-sized chunks, place in a roasting tin with the onion and garlic and drizzle with the oil. Season and bake for 1 hour, or until the vegetables are tender. Leave to cool.

3 Mix the flours, margarine and ricotta cheese in a food processor, then slowly add up to 3 tablespoons of the milk, or enough to form a soft dough. Turn out onto a lightly floured surface and gather together into a smooth ball. Cover and refrigerate for 15 minutes.

4 Roll the pastry out on a lightly floured surface, then ease into the tin, bringing it gently up the side of the tin. Trim the edge and refrigerate for 10 minutes. Increase the oven to 200°C (400°F/Gas 6). Cover the pastry with crumpled baking paper and fill with baking beads or uncooked rice. Bake for 10 minutes, remove the beads and paper, then bake for another 10 minutes, or until golden brown.

5 Place the vegetables in the pastry base and pour in the combined remaining milk, eggs, cheese and basil. Reduce the oven to 180°C (350°F/Gas 4) and bake for 1 hour 10 minutes, or until set in the centre. Leave for 5 minutes before removing from the tin to serve.

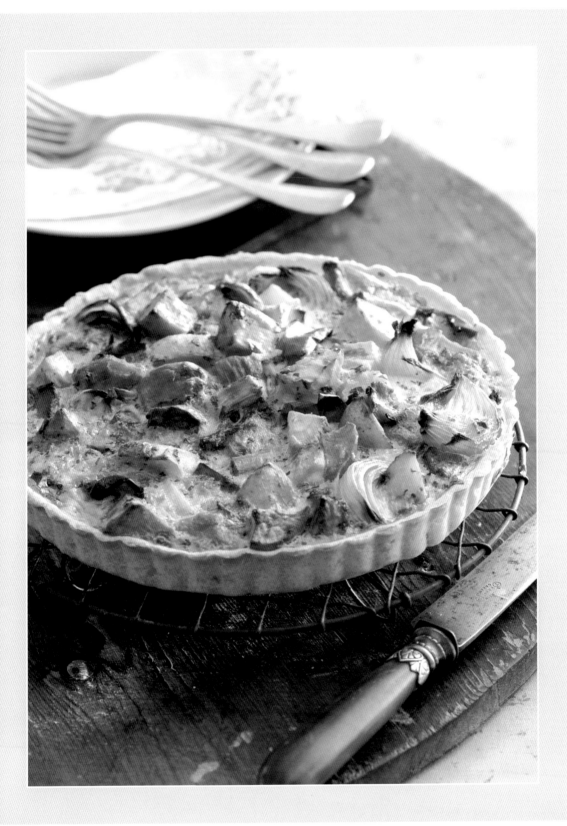

Vegetarian rice paper rolls

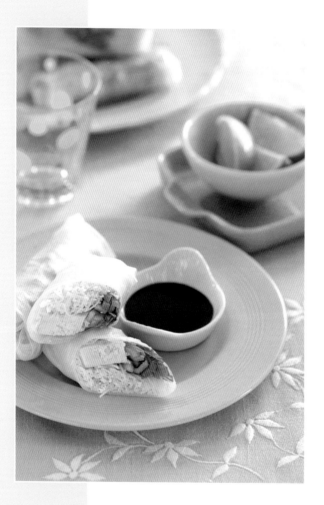

50 g (1¾ oz) dried rice vermicelli

200 g (7 oz) frozen soya beans

16 square (15 cm/6 in) rice paper
   wrappers

1 zucchini (courgette), cut into
   thin matchsticks

1 Lebanese (short) cucumber,
   cut into thin matchsticks

1 carrot, grated

1 large handful mint, finely shredded

100 g (3½ oz) firm tofu, cut into
   1 cm (½ in) wide batons

nutrition per serve
Energy **1284 kJ (307 Cal)** Fat **5.7 g** Saturated fat **0.7 g**
Protein **15.1 g** Carbohydrate **46.5 g** Fibre **5 g** Cholesterol **0 mg** Sodium **1654 mg**

Dipping sauce

80 ml (2½ fl oz/⅓ cup) fish sauce

2 tbsp chopped coriander (cilantro)
   leaves

2 small red chillies, finely chopped

2 tsp soft brown sugar

2 tsp lime juice

Prep time 40 minutes +
5 minutes soaking

Cooking time 2 minutes

Serves 4

1 Soak the vermicelli in hot water for 5 minutes, or until soft. Drain and cut into 5 cm (2 in) lengths using scissors. Bring a saucepan of water to the boil, add the soya beans and cook for 2 minutes, then drain well.

2 Working with two wrappers at a time, dip each rice paper wrapper in warm water for 10 seconds. Remove from the water and lay out on a flat work surface.

3 Place a small amount of vermicelli noodles on the bottom third of each wrapper, leaving a 2 cm (¾ in) border either side. Top with some zucchini, cucumber, carrot, soya beans, mint and two batons of tofu. Keeping the filling compact and neat, fold in the sides and roll up tightly. Seal with a little water. Cover with a damp cloth while you assemble the remaining rolls.

4 To make the dipping sauce, combine the fish sauce, coriander, chilli, sugar, lime juice and 2 tablespoons water in a small bowl. Serve with the rice paper rolls.

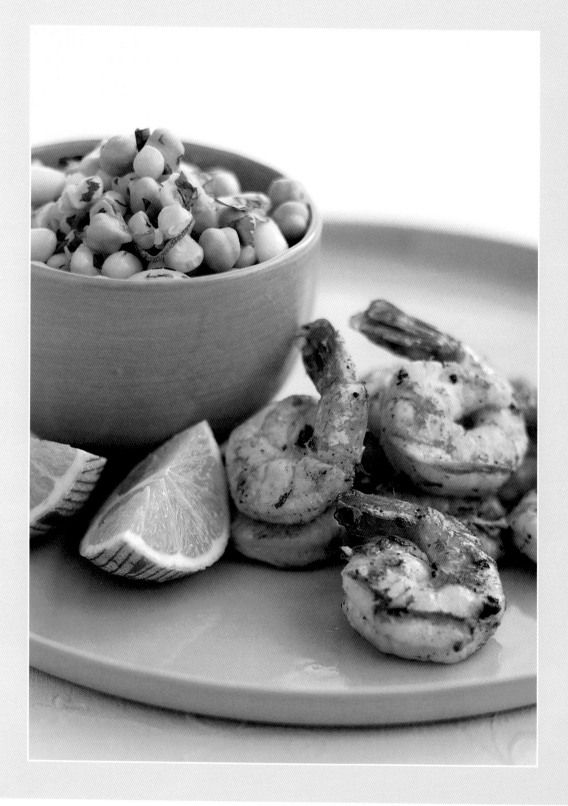

Prawns with corn salsa

**400 g (14 oz) tin cannellini beans,
drained and rinsed**

**300 g (10½ oz) tin chickpeas,
drained and rinsed**

**310 g (11 oz) tin corn kernels,
drained and rinsed**

1 tsp grated lime zest

**2 tbsp chopped coriander (cilantro)
leaves**

**500 g (1 lb 2 oz) large raw prawns
(shrimp)**

2 tbsp lemon juice

1 tbsp sesame oil

2 garlic cloves, crushed

2 tsp grated fresh ginger

canola or olive oil spray

lime wedges, to serve

1 Combine the cannellini beans, chickpeas and corn kernels in a large bowl. Stir in the lime zest and coriander.

2 Peel the prawns, leaving the tails intact. Gently pull out the dark vein from each prawn back, starting at the head end.

3 To make the marinade, combine the lemon juice, sesame oil, garlic and ginger in a small bowl. Add the prawns and gently stir to coat them in the marinade. Cover and refrigerate for at least 3 hours.

4 Lightly spray a barbecue hotplate with oil and heat to high. Add the prawns and cook for 3–5 minutes, or until pink and cooked through. Brush frequently with the marinade while cooking. Serve immediately with the corn, bean and chickpea salsa and wedges of lime.

Prep time 15 minutes +
3 hours marinating
Cooking time 5 minutes
Serves 4

nutrition per serve   Energy **1338 kJ (320 Cal)** Fat **15.1 g** Saturated fat **3.6 g**
Protein **6.7 g** Carbohydrate **36.5 g** Fibre **5.7 g** Cholesterol **6 mg** Sodium **101 mg**

Sweet potatoes with salsa

4 x 200 g (7 oz) orange sweet
   potatoes, unpeeled

1 red onion, finely chopped

1 avocado, finely chopped

1 tbsp lemon juice

125 g (4½ oz) tin corn kernels,
   drained and rinsed

½ red capsicum (pepper), finely
   chopped

1 tbsp sweet chilli sauce

2 tbsp light sour cream or low-fat
   plain yoghurt

2 tbsp chopped flat-leaf (Italian)
   parsley

1 Preheat the oven to 200°C (400°F/Gas 6). Scrub the
    sweet potatoes clean, dry them and pierce several
    times with a skewer. Bake directly on the oven rack for
    40 minutes, or until tender when tested with a skewer.

2 Meanwhile, put the onion, avocado, lemon juice, corn
    and capsicum in a bowl and mix together well. Stir in
    the chilli sauce and season with salt (if desired) and
    freshly ground black pepper.

3 Make a deep cut along the top of each cooked sweet
    potato. Divide the topping among the sweet potatoes
    and add a dollop of sour cream or yoghurt to each.
    Sprinkle with the parsley and serve with a green salad.

Prep time 15 minutes

Cooking time 40 minutes

Serves 4

nutrition per serve Energy **585 kJ (140 Cal)** Fat **4 g** Saturated fat **0.5 g**
Protein **8.8 g** Carbohydrate **14.9 g** Fibre **5.3 g** Cholesterol **0 mg** Sodium **7 mg**

Dal

200 g (7 oz/1 cup) red lentils

¼ tsp ground turmeric

1 tbsp oil

½ tsp brown mustard seeds

1 tbsp cumin seeds

1 onion, finely chopped

1 tbsp grated fresh ginger

2 long green chillies, halved lengthways

80 ml (2½ fl oz/⅓ cup) lemon juice

2 tbsp finely chopped coriander (cilantro) leaves

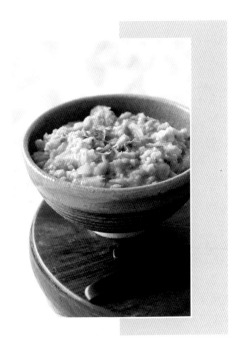

1 Put the lentils in a saucepan, cover with 750 ml (26 fl oz/3 cups) water and bring to the boil. Reduce the heat, stir in the turmeric, then cover and simmer for 20 minutes, or until the lentils are tender.

2 Heat the oil in a saucepan, add the mustard and cumin seeds and cook until the mustard seeds begin to pop. Add the onion, ginger and chillies and cook for 5 minutes, or until the onion is golden.

3 Add the lentils and 125 ml (4 fl oz/½ cup) water to the pan. Season with salt (if desired), reduce the heat and simmer for 10 minutes. Remove from the heat, stir in the lemon juice and garnish with the coriander. Serve with naan breads, or as part of a vegetarian meal with rice and curried vegetables.

Prep time 10 minutes
Cooking time 40 minutes
Serves 6

nutrition per serve Energy **1309 kJ (313 Cal)** Fat **14.8 g** Saturated fat **4.8 g**
Protein **19.1 g** Carbohydrate **23.2 g** Fibre **7.4 g** Cholesterol **260 mg** Sodium **487 mg**

Vegetable frittata

2 large red capsicums (peppers)

500 g (1 lb 2 oz) eggplant (aubergine),
   cut into 1 cm (½ in) slices

olive oil spray

600 g (1 lb 5 oz) orange sweet potato,
   peeled and cut into 1 cm (½ in)
   slices

2 tsp olive oil

2 leeks, white part only, thinly sliced

2 garlic cloves, crushed

250 g (9 oz) zucchini (courgette),
   thinly sliced

8 eggs, lightly beaten

2 tbsp finely chopped basil

70 g (2½ oz/¾ cup) grated parmesan
   cheese

200 g (7 oz) reduced-fat hummus

baby rocket (arugula) leaves, to serve

Prep time 30 minutes
Cooking time 40 minutes
Serves 6

1 Cut the capsicums into large flat pieces, removing the seeds and membranes. Put the capsicums, skin side up, under a preheated grill (broiler) until the skin blackens. Leave covered under a tea towel (dish towel) until cool, then peel away the skin.

2 Arrange the eggplant slices in a single layer on the grill tray. Spray with oil and grill (broil) for 2–3 minutes. Turn the eggplant slices over and respray with oil, cooking for a further 2–3 minutes, or until softened. Drain on paper towels.

3 Cook the sweet potato in a saucepan of boiling water for 4–5 minutes, or until just tender, then drain well.

4 Heat the oil in a deep round 23 cm (9 in) frying pan over medium heat. Add the leek and garlic and stir for 1 minute, or until soft. Add the zucchini and cook for 2 minutes, then remove from the pan.

5 Line the base of the pan with half the eggplant and top with the leek mixture. Cover with the roasted capsicum, then with the remaining eggplant and finally the sweet potato.

6 Put the eggs, basil and parmesan in a bowl and season with freshly ground black pepper. Mix well and pour over the vegetables in the pan. Cook over low heat for 15 minutes, or until almost cooked. Place the pan under a hot grill for 2–3 minutes, or until the top of the frittata is golden and cooked. Cut into six wedges. Serve with hummus and rocket.

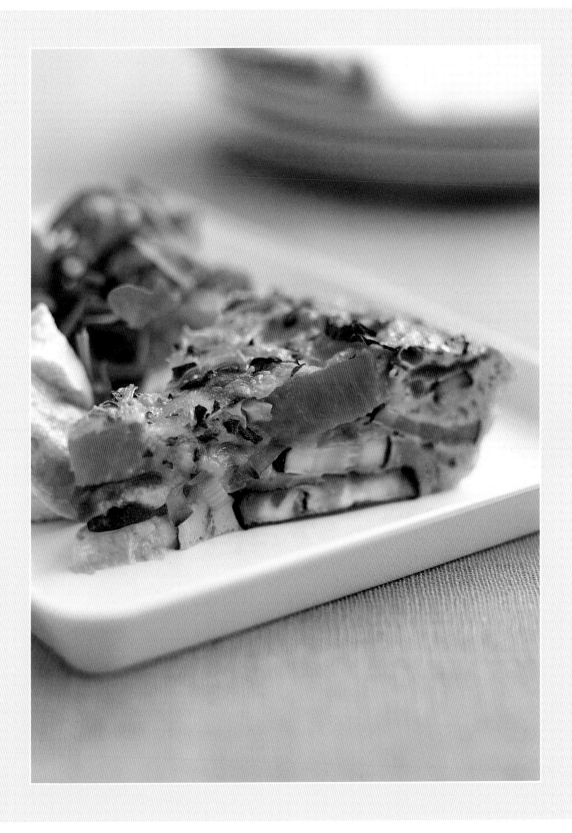

Beef pittas with salsa

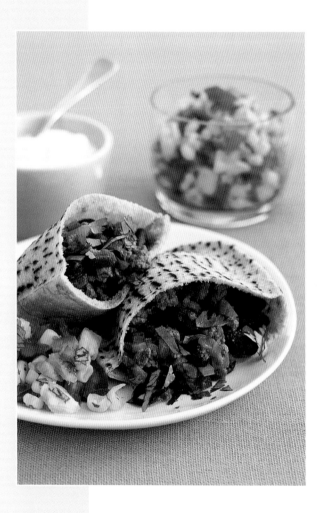

1 tsp olive oil

1 onion, finely chopped

1 celery stalk, finely chopped

½ red capsicum (pepper), finely chopped

400 g (14 oz) lean minced (ground) beef

1 tsp ground cumin

½ tsp ground coriander

1 tbsp tomato paste (concentrated purée)

250 g (9 oz/1 cup) bottled tomato pasta sauce

240 g (8½ oz) tinned red kidney beans, drained and rinsed

4 wholemeal (whole-wheat) pitta breads

250 g (9 oz/1 cup) low-fat plain yoghurt

Pineapple salsa

½ **pineapple**

4 **vine-ripened tomatoes**

310 g (11 oz) **tin corn kernels,
drained and rinsed**

50 g (1¾ oz/½ **large bunch)
coriander (cilantro) leaves,
chopped**

1 tbsp **lemon juice**

Prep time 15 minutes
Cooking time 20 minutes
Serves 4

1 Heat the oil in a large, non-stick frying pan. Add the onion, celery and capsicum and cook, stirring, for 2 minutes, or until softened. Increase the heat, add the beef and cook for 5 minutes, or until the meat changes colour. Break up any lumps with a fork. Stir in the cumin, ground coriander and tomato paste. Add the pasta sauce and 125 ml (4 fl oz/½ cup) water. Simmer and stir frequently for 8 minutes, or until cooked and slightly reduced. Stir in the kidney beans.

2 To make the pineapple salsa, peel and finely chop the pineapple. Cut the tomatoes into quarters, remove the seeds with a spoon, and finely chop the flesh. Combine the salsa ingredients, reserving half of the coriander leaves for garnish.

3 Preheat the oven to 180°C (350°F/Gas 4). Wrap the pitta breads in foil and warm them in the oven for 5 minutes.

4 To serve, cut the pitta breads in half, fill with the beef and bean mixture and top with the yoghurt. Sprinkle with the reserved coriander and serve with the salsa.

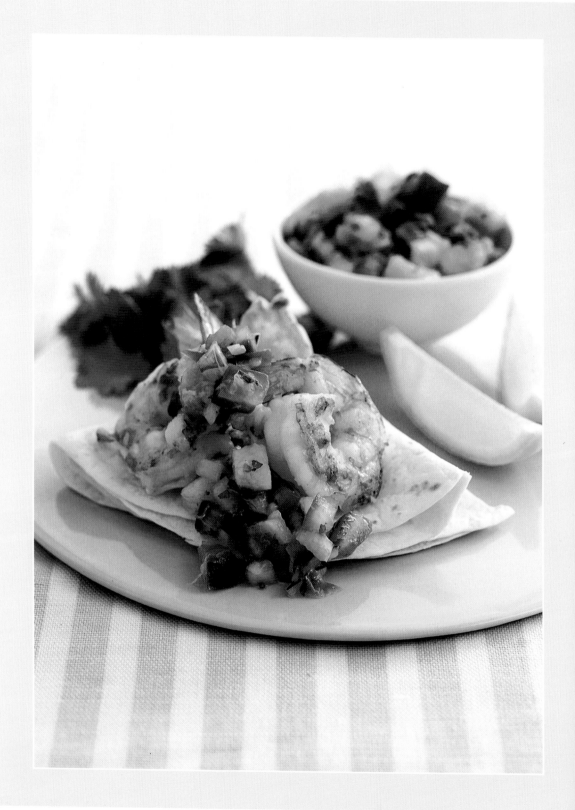

Prawn tortillas with mango salsa

Mango salsa

½ red onion, finely chopped

2 mangoes, finely chopped

4 vine-ripened tomatoes, seeded and finely chopped

1 Lebanese (short) cucumber, peeled, seeded and finely chopped

1 celery stalk, thinly sliced

3 handfuls mint, chopped

2 tbsp fat-free French dressing

olive oil spray

16 raw prawns (shrimp), peeled and deveined, tails left intact

8 flour tortillas (20 cm/8 in)

coriander (cilantro) leaves, to serve

lemon wedges, to serve

1 To make the mango salsa, combine the onion, mango, tomato, cucumber, celery and mint in a large bowl. Add the dressing and toss to combine.

2 Lightly spray a barbecue hotplate with the oil and heat to high. Add the prawns and cook, turning occasionally, for 2–3 minutes, or until just cooked through. Wrap the tortillas in foil and place them on a warm part of the barbecue to heat through.

3 To serve, fold the tortillas into four. Arrange the tortillas, mango salsa and prawns on the plate and garnish with the coriander leaves. Serve with the lemon wedges.

Prep time 20 minutes
Cooking time 5 minutes
Makes 8

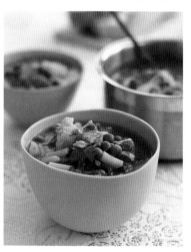 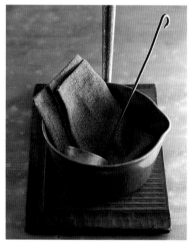 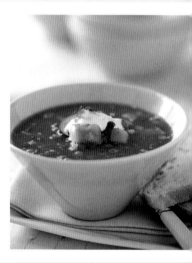

Soups

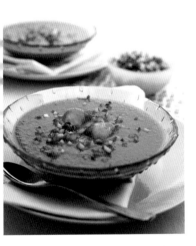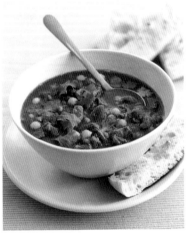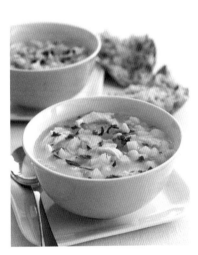

nutrition per serve   Energy **1140 kJ (272 Cal)** Fat **9.6 g** Saturated fat **2.3 g** Protein **15.2 g** Carbohydrate **26.9 g** Fibre **11.3 g** Cholesterol **20 mg**   Sodium **970 mg**

Lentil and vegetable soup

2 tbsp olive oil

1 small leek, white part only, chopped

2 garlic cloves, crushed

2 tsp curry powder

1 tsp ground cumin

1 tsp garam masala

1 litre (35 fl oz/4 cups) vegetable stock

1 bay leaf

185 g (6½ oz/1 cup) brown lentils

450 g (1 lb) butternut pumpkin (squash), peeled and cut into 1 cm (½ in) cubes

2 zucchini (courgettes), cut in half lengthways and sliced

400 g (14 oz) tin chopped tomatoes

200 g (7 oz) broccoli, cut into small florets

1 small carrot, diced

80 g (2¾ oz/½ cup) peas

1 tbsp chopped mint

Spiced yoghurt

250 g (9 oz/1 cup) Greek-style yoghurt

1 tbsp chopped coriander (cilantro) leaves

1 garlic clove, crushed

3 dashes Tabasco sauce

1 Heat the olive oil in a saucepan over medium heat, add the leek and garlic and cook for 4–5 minutes, or until soft and lightly golden. Add the curry powder, cumin and garam masala and cook for 1 minute, or until fragrant.

2 Add the stock, bay leaf, lentils and pumpkin. Bring to the boil, then reduce the heat to low and simmer for 10–15 minutes, or until the lentils are tender. Season well.

3 Add the zucchini, tomatoes, broccoli, carrot and 500 ml (17 fl oz/2 cups) water and simmer for 10 minutes, or until the vegetables are tender. Add the peas and simmer for a further 2–3 minutes.

4 To make the spiced yoghurt, put the yoghurt, coriander, garlic and Tabasco in a small bowl and stir until combined. Dollop a spoonful of the yoghurt on each serving of soup and garnish with the chopped mint.

Prep time 20 minutes

Cooking time 35 minutes

Serves 6

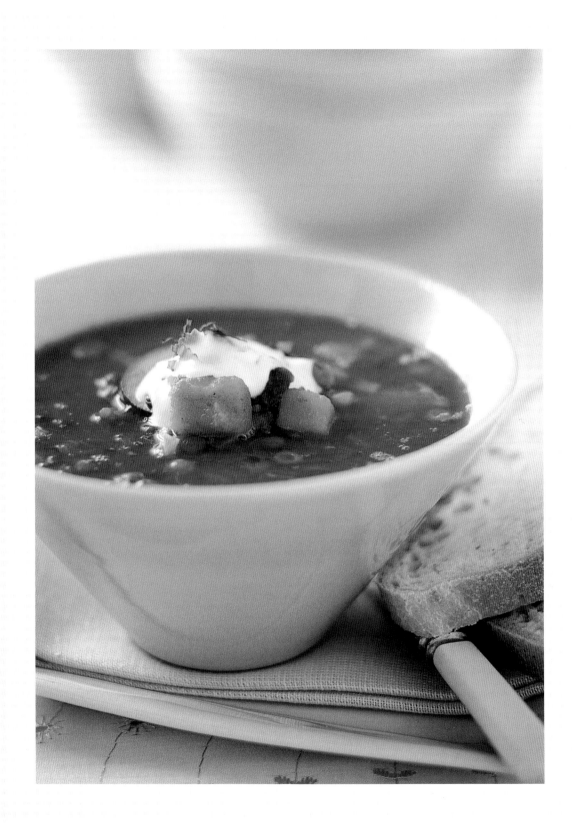

nutrition per serve (8) Energy **998 kJ (239 Cal)** Fat **6.1 g** Saturated fat **0.8 g**
Protein **14.7 g** Carbohydrate **28.4 g** Fibre **6.5 g** Cholesterol **0 mg** Sodium **561 mg**

Split pea soup

2 tbsp olive oil

1 large onion, chopped

1 large carrot, cut into 1 cm
    (½ in) cubes

1 large celery stalk, cut into
    1 cm (½ in) cubes

2 bay leaves

1 tbsp thyme, finely chopped

6 garlic cloves, finely chopped

440 g (15½ oz/2 cups) yellow
    split peas

1 litre (35 fl oz/4 cups) chicken stock

3 tbsp lemon juice

olive oil, extra, to serve

1 Heat the oil in a large saucepan over medium heat. Add the onion, carrot and celery and cook for 4–5 minutes, or until starting to brown. Add the bay leaves, thyme and garlic and cook for 1 minute.

2 Stir in the split peas, then add the stock and 1 litre (35 fl oz/4 cups) water. Cook for 1 hour 15 minutes, or until the split peas and vegetables are soft. Stir often during cooking to prevent the soup from sticking to the bottom of the pan, and skim any scum from the surface. Add a little extra water if the soup is too thick.

3 Remove from the heat and discard the bay leaves. Stir in the lemon juice and season with salt (if desired) and freshly ground black pepper. Drizzle with a little olive oil before serving.

Prep time 20 minutes

Cooking time 1 hour 20 minutes

Serves 6–8

nutrition per serve Energy **1783 kJ (426 Cal)** Fat **17 g** Saturated fat **5.9 g**
Protein **41.2 g** Carbohydrate **22.5 g** Fibre **8 g** Cholesterol **77 mg** Sodium **2761 mg**

Beef and chilli bean soup

1 tbsp olive oil

1 red onion, finely chopped

2 garlic cloves, crushed

2½ tsp chilli flakes

2½ tsp ground cumin

1½ tsp ground coriander

2½ tbsp finely chopped coriander
(cilantro) root and stem

500 g (1 lb 2 oz) lean minced
(ground) beef

2 litres (70 fl oz/8 cups) beef stock

4 tomatoes, seeded and diced

1 tbsp tomato paste (concentrated
purée)

420 g (15 oz) tin red kidney beans,
drained and rinsed

3 tbsp chopped coriander (cilantro)
leaves

90 g (3¼ oz/⅓ cup) light sour cream

Prep time 20 minutes
Cooking time 30 minutes
Serves 4

1 Heat the oil in a large saucepan over medium heat and cook the onion for 2–3 minutes, or until softened. Add the garlic, chilli flakes, ground cumin, ground coriander and coriander root and stem and cook for another minute. Add the beef and cook for 3–4 minutes, or until cooked through, breaking up any lumps with the back of a wooden spoon.

2 Add the stock, tomatoes, tomato paste and kidney beans and bring to the boil over high heat. Reduce the heat and simmer for 15–20 minutes, or until reduced slightly. Remove any scum that rises to the surface. Stir in the coriander leaves and season with salt (if desired) and freshly ground black pepper. Divide among four serving bowls and top with a dollop of sour cream.

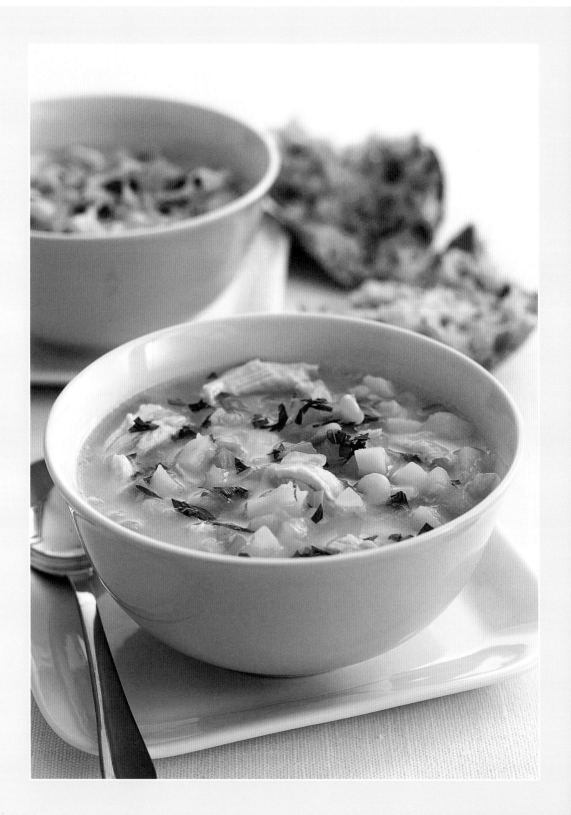

nutrition per serve   Energy **1285 kJ (307 Cal)** Fat **2.3 g** Saturated fat **0.6 g**
Protein **21.4 g** Carbohydrate **45.5 g** Fibre **8.1 g** Cholesterol **33 mg** Sodium **1547 mg**

Chicken corn chowder

180 g (6 oz) boneless skinless
   chicken breast, trimmed

1 litre (35 fl oz/4 cups) chicken stock
   or water

1 large onion, diced

2 potatoes, diced

1 celery stalk, diced

1 large carrot, grated

420 g (15 oz) tin creamed corn

310 g (11 oz) tin corn kernels,
   drained and rinsed

125 ml (4 fl oz/½ cup) skim or no-fat
   milk

3 tbsp finely chopped flat-leaf
   (Italian) parsley

1 Cut 2–3 slits across the thickest part of the chicken.
Heat the stock in a large heavy-based saucepan, add the
chicken and poach for 10 minutes, or until just cooked
through. Remove the chicken from the pan and set
aside. When cooled, use two forks to thinly shred the
chicken flesh.

2 Add the onion, potato, celery and carrot to the
saucepan. Bring to the boil, then lower the heat and
simmer for 20 minutes, or until the potato is cooked.

3 Stir in the chicken, creamed corn, corn kernels, milk
and parsley. Stir gently to heat through and serve.

Prep time 15 minutes

Cooking time 35 minutes

Serves 4

nutrition per serve Energy **1359 kJ (325 Cal)** Fat **12 g** Saturated fat **1.6 g**
Protein **10.3 g** Carbohydrate **39 g** Fibre **7.6 g** Cholesterol **0 mg** Sodium **755 mg**

Gazpacho

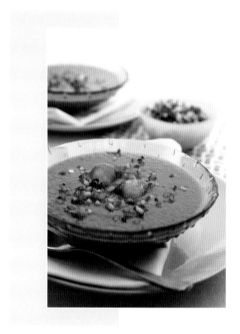

Prep time 20 minutes
Cooking time Nil
Serves 4

1 kg (2 lb 4 oz) vine-ripened tomatoes

½ telegraph (long) cucumber, roughly chopped

4 spring onions (scallions), thinly sliced

1 red capsicum (pepper), roughly chopped

2 garlic cloves, crushed

250 ml (9 fl oz/1 cup) chilled chicken stock

2 tbsp extra virgin olive oil

3 tbsp red wine vinegar

1 slice day-old Italian-style bread, roughly torn

1 small handful basil, shredded

40 g (1½ oz/⅓ cup) pitted black olives, sliced

4 wholegrain bread rolls, to serve

1 To peel the tomatoes, score a cross in the base of each tomato. Put in a heatproof bowl and cover with boiling water. Leave for 30 seconds, then transfer to cold water and peel the skin away from the cross. Roughly cut into quarters.

2 Place the tomatoes in a large bowl and add the cucumber, spring onion, capsicum, garlic, stock, oil, vinegar and bread. Mix well.

3 Process the mixture in a blender or food processor in batches, taking care to add enough of the liquid so the mixture blends easily. Thin the soup with water or more stock if desired. Season to taste with salt (if desired) and freshly ground black pepper and serve chilled, garnished with the basil and olives. Serve with the bread rolls.

nutrition per serve   Energy 1812 kJ (433 Cal) Fat 11.6 g Saturated fat 4.1 g
Protein 36.2 g Carbohydrate 35.3 g Fibre 6.6 g Cholesterol 84 mg Sodium 2299 mg

Winter lamb shank soup

1 tbsp olive oil

1.25 kg (2 lb 12 oz) trimmed
    lamb shanks

2 onions, chopped

4 garlic cloves, chopped

250 ml (9 fl oz/1 cup) red wine

2 bay leaves

1 tbsp chopped rosemary

2.5 litres (87 fl oz/10 cups) beef stock

400 g (14 oz) tin crushed tomatoes

165 g (5¾ oz/¾ cup) pearl barley,
    rinsed and drained

1 large carrot, unpeeled, diced

1 potato, unpeeled, diced

1 turnip, peeled and diced

1 parsnip, peeled and diced

2 tbsp redcurrant jelly (optional)

Prep time 30 minutes
Cooking time 4 hours
Serves 6

1   Heat the oil in a large saucepan or stockpot over high
    heat. Add the shanks and cook for 2–3 minutes, or until
    browned. Remove and set aside.

2   Add the onion to the pan and cook over low heat for
    8 minutes, or until softened. Add the garlic and cook for
    a further 30 seconds, then add the wine and simmer for
    5 minutes, scraping up any sediment stuck to the
    bottom of the pan.

3   Return the shanks to the pan along with the bay leaves
    and half the rosemary. Pour in 1.5 litres (52 fl oz/6 cups)
    of the stock and then season with salt (if desired) and
    pepper. Bring to the boil over high heat, then reduce the
    heat and simmer, covered, for 2 hours, or until the meat
    is falling off the bones.

4   Remove the shanks and cool slightly. Remove the meat
    from the bones and roughly chop. Add the meat to the
    broth along with the tomatoes, barley and remaining
    rosemary and stock. Simmer for 30 minutes. Add the
    vegetables and cook for 1 hour, or until the barley is
    tender. Remove the bay leaves and stir in the redcurrant
    jelly, if using. Serve immediately.

nutrition per serve (6)   Energy **1060 kJ (253 Cal)** Fat **4.2 g** Saturated fat **1.2 g**
Protein **17.6 g** Carbohydrate **32.4 g** Fibre **8.5 g** Cholesterol **16 mg** Sodium **2002 mg**

Hearty bean and vegetable soup

1 tsp olive oil

100 g (3½ oz) pancetta, trimmed
   and diced

1 leek, white part only, thinly sliced

2 garlic cloves, chopped

1 celery stalk, thinly sliced

1 large carrot, diced

2 waxy potatoes, diced

2 litres (70 fl oz/8 cups)
   chicken stock

400 g (14 oz) tin chopped tomatoes

80 g (2¾ oz/½ cup) macaroni

155 g (5½ oz/1 cup) frozen peas,
   thawed

1 zucchini (courgette), thinly sliced

185 g (6½ oz) cauliflower, cut into
   small florets

400 g (14 oz) tin cannellini beans,
   drained and rinsed

1 handful flat-leaf (Italian) parsley,
   chopped

grated parmesan cheese, to serve
   (optional)

1 Heat the oil in a large saucepan over low heat. Add
the pancetta, leek and garlic and cook, stirring, for
10 minutes, without browning. Add the celery, carrot
and potato. Cook for a further 5 minutes, stirring.

2 Pour in the stock and add the tomatoes. Bring slowly
to the boil, then reduce the heat and simmer for
15 minutes. Stir in the pasta, peas, zucchini, cauliflower
and cannellini beans. Simmer for a further 10 minutes,
or until the pasta is cooked.

3 Before serving, stir in the parsley. Serve with grated
parmesan, if desired, and crusty wholegrain bread.

Prep time 25 minutes

Cooking time 40 minutes

Serves 4–6

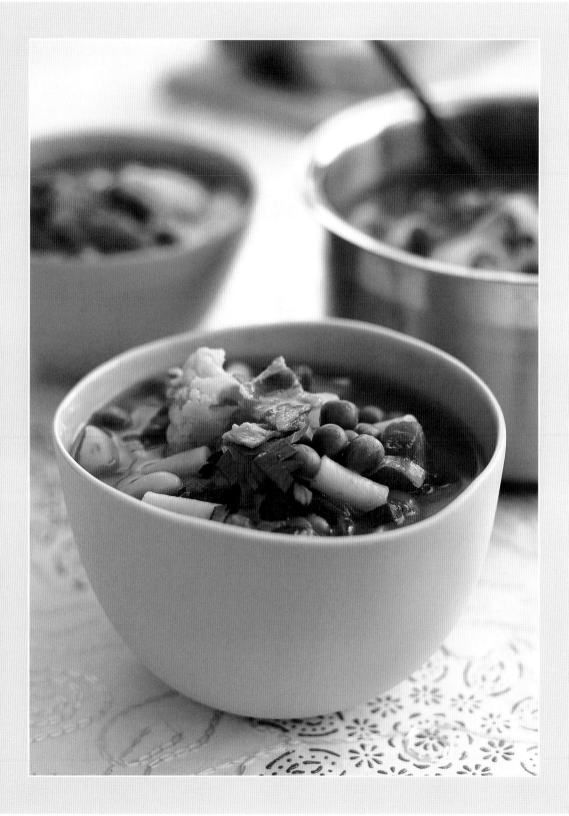

nutrition per serve (6)   Energy **757 kJ (181 Cal)** Fat **4.6 g** Saturated fat **0.8 g**
Protein **8.6 g** Carbohydrate **23 g** Fibre **7 g** Cholesterol **3 mg** Sodium **1366 mg**

Roasted vegetable soup

750 g (1 lb 10 oz) unpeeled carrots, chopped into 5 cm (2 in) pieces

350 g (12 oz) unpeeled orange sweet potato, chopped into 5 cm (2 in) pieces

2 zucchini (courgettes), halved lengthways

1 tbsp olive oil

2 onions, cut into wedges

3 unpeeled garlic cloves

1 bay leaf

4 parsley stalks

2 thyme sprigs

1.5 litres (52 fl oz/6 cups) chicken stock

400 g (14 oz) tin chopped tomatoes

1 tbsp tomato paste (concentrated purée)

4 thin slices pancetta or prosciutto, chopped

1 Preheat the oven to 180°C (350°F/Gas 4). Put the carrot, sweet potato and zucchini in a large shallow roasting tin. Drizzle with the oil and toss to coat the vegetables. Bake for 30 minutes, then add the onion and garlic. Bake for a further 30 minutes, or until the vegetables are tender and lightly browned. Turn the vegetables occasionally during baking. Peel the garlic cloves.

2 Transfer the garlic and the contents of the roasting tin to a large saucepan. Tie the bay leaf, parsley stalks and thyme sprigs together and add to the pan. Add the stock, tomatoes and tomato paste. Bring to the boil, then reduce the heat and simmer for 20 minutes. Cool for 10 minutes, then remove the bay leaf, parsley and thyme sprigs. Use a potato masher to roughly mash the vegetables. Season with salt (if desired) and freshly ground black pepper.

3 Heat a small frying pan over medium heat, add the pancetta and cook until crisp. Reheat the soup just before serving and sprinkle over the crumbled pancetta. Serve with crunchy wholegrain bread or toast.

Prep time 20 minutes
Cooking time 1½ hours
Serves 4–6

nutrition per serve   Energy **1827 kJ (436 Cal)** Fat **6.9 g** Saturated fat **1.2 g**
Protein **38.4 g** Carbohydrate **47 g** Fibre **11.8 g** Cholesterol **51 mg** Sodium **1389 mg**

Mediterranean fish soup

$^1\!/_2$ **tsp saffron threads**

2 tsp olive oil

1 large onion, thinly sliced

1 leek, white part only, chopped

4 garlic cloves, finely chopped

$^1\!/_2$ **tsp dried oregano**

1 tsp grated orange zest

2 tbsp dry white wine

**1 red capsicum (pepper), cut into
    bite-sized pieces**

2 zucchini (courgettes), chopped

**500 g (1 lb 2 oz) ripe tomatoes,
    chopped**

**125 ml (4 fl oz/$^1\!/_2$ cup) tomato
    passata (puréed tomatoes)**

750 ml (26 fl oz/3 cups) fish stock

**2 tbsp tomato paste (concentrated
    purée)**

2 tsp soft brown sugar

**500 g (1 lb 2 oz) skinless and
    boneless fish fillets, trimmed and
    cut into bite-sized pieces**

**300 g (10$^1\!/_2$ oz) tin red kidney beans,
    drained and rinsed**

4 tbsp chopped parsley

4 wholegrain bread rolls

1   Soak the saffron threads in a small bowl with
2 tablespoons boiling water.

2   Heat the oil in a large saucepan over low heat. Add
the onion, leek, garlic and oregano. Cover and cook for
10 minutes, shaking the pan occasionally, until the
onion is soft. Add the orange zest, wine, capsicum,
zucchini and tomatoes, cover and cook for 10 minutes.

3   Add the tomato passata, stock, tomato paste, sugar and
saffron (along with the soaking water) to the pan. Stir
well and bring to the boil, then reduce the heat to low
and simmer, uncovered, for 15 minutes.

4   Add the fish to the soup, cover and cook for 8 minutes,
or until tender. Add the kidney beans and half the
parsley and season to taste with salt (if desired) and
freshly ground black pepper. Sprinkle the soup with the
remaining parsley just before serving. Serve with bread
rolls.

Prep time 30 minutes
Cooking time 45 minutes
Serves 4

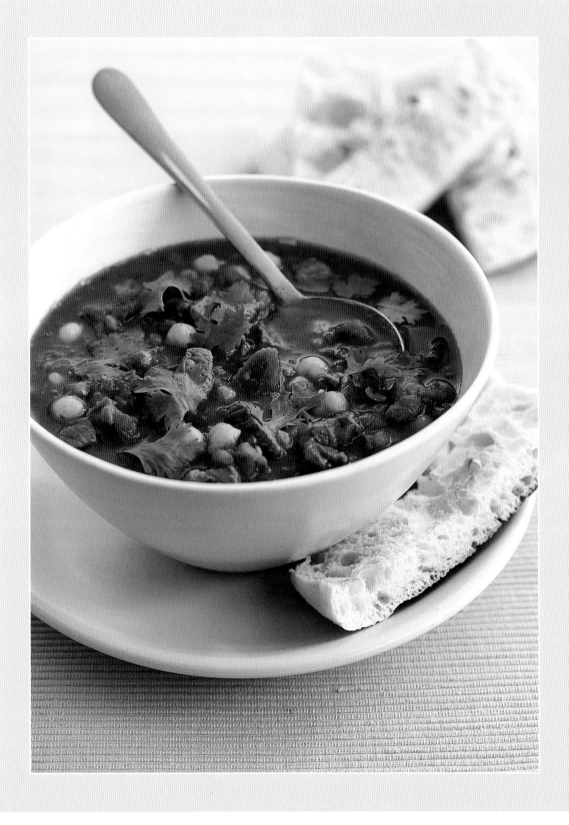

nutrition per serve (6)   Energy **1877 kJ (448 Cal)** Fat **14.2 g** Saturated fat **4.9 g**
Protein **45.8 g** Carbohydrate **28 g** Fibre **10.1 g** Cholesterol **96 mg** Sodium **104 mg**

Moroccan lamb soup

165 g (5¾ oz/¾ cup) dried chickpeas

1 tbsp olive oil

850 g (1 lb 14 oz) boned lamb leg,
 cut into 1 cm (½ in) cubes

1 onion, chopped

2 garlic cloves, crushed

½ tsp ground cinnamon

½ tsp ground turmeric

½ tsp ground ginger

4 tbsp chopped coriander (cilantro)
 leaves

2 x 400 g (14 oz) tins diced tomatoes

1 litre (35 fl oz/4 cups) chicken stock

135 g (4¾ oz/⅔ cup) red lentils

fresh coriander (cilantro) leaves,
 to garnish

Turkish bread, to serve

Prep time 15 minutes +
overnight soaking
Cooking time 2¼ hours
Serves 4–6

1 Put the chickpeas in a large bowl, cover with water and soak overnight. Drain and rinse under cold water and drain again.

2 Heat the oil in a large saucepan over high heat. Add the lamb and brown in batches for 2–3 minutes. Reduce the heat to medium, return all the lamb to the pan along with the onion and garlic and cook for 5 minutes. Add the cinnamon, turmeric, ginger, a pinch of salt (if desired) and 1 teaspoon freshly ground black pepper and cook for a further 2 minutes. Add the chopped coriander, tomatoes, stock and 500 ml (17 fl oz/2 cups) water and bring to the boil over high heat.

3 Rinse the lentils under cold water and drain. Add the lentils and chickpeas to the pan, then reduce the heat and simmer, covered, for 1½ hours. Uncover and cook for a further 30 minutes, or until the lamb is tender and the soup is thick. Season to taste. Divide the soup among serving bowls and garnish with the coriander leaves. Serve with toasted Turkish bread.

nutrition per serve (6) Energy **1554 kJ (371 Cal)** Fat **8.2 g** Saturated fat **1.3 g**
Protein **24.7 g** Carbohydrate **44.5 g** Fibre **12.5 g** Cholesterol **1 mg** Sodium **1664 mg**

Red lentil, burghul and mint soup

2 tomatoes, finely chopped

2 tbsp olive oil

1 large red onion, finely chopped

2 garlic cloves, crushed

2 tbsp tomato paste (concentrated purée)

2 tsp ground paprika

½ tsp cayenne pepper

400 g (14 oz/2 cups) red lentils

50 g (1¾ oz/¼ cup) basmati rice

2.125 litres (74 fl oz/8½ cups) chicken stock

50 g (1¾ oz/¼ cup) fine burghul (bulgur)

2 tbsp chopped mint

2 tbsp chopped flat-leaf (Italian) parsley

90 g (3¼ oz/⅓ cup) low-fat plain yoghurt

¼ preserved lemon, pulp removed, rind washed and cut into thin strips

1 To peel the tomatoes, score a cross in the base of each tomato. Put in a heatproof bowl and cover with boiling water. Leave for 30 seconds, then transfer to cold water and peel skin away from the cross. Finely chop the flesh.

2 Heat the oil in a large saucepan over medium heat. Add the onion and garlic and cook for 2–3 minutes, or until soft. Stir in the tomatoes, tomato paste, paprika and cayenne pepper and cook for 1 minute.

3 Add the lentils, rice and stock, cover and bring to the boil over high heat. Reduce the heat and simmer for 30–35 minutes, or until the rice is cooked.

4 Stir in the burghul, mint and parsley and season with salt (if desired) and freshly ground black pepper. Divide the soup among serving bowls and garnish with the yoghurt and preserved lemon. Serve immediately.

Prep time 25 minutes
Cooking time 45 minutes
Serves 4–6

Pea and ham soup

440 g (15½ oz/2 cups) split green peas, rinsed and drained

750 g (1 lb 10 oz) ham bones

1 celery stalk, including leaves, chopped

1 carrot, diced

1 onion, chopped

3 leeks, sliced

1 orange sweet potato, peeled and chopped

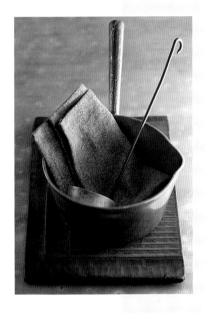

1 Put the split peas in a large bowl, cover with water and leave to soak for at least 4 hours or overnight. Drain and rinse well.

2 Put the ham bones, split peas, celery, carrot and onion in a large saucepan with 2.5 litres (87 fl oz/10 cups) water. Bring to the boil, then reduce the heat and simmer, covered, for 2 hours, or until the split peas are very soft.

3 Add the leek and sweet potato to the pan and cook for 30 minutes, or until the vegetables are tender and the ham is falling off the bone. Remove the ham bones from the soup, cut off all the meat and finely chop.

4 Transfer the soup to a bowl to cool, then use a potato masher to lightly mash—the soup should be chunky. Return the soup to the pan, stir in the chopped ham and reheat the soup to serve. Either serve the soup on its own as a starter, or serve with toasted wholegrain bread and salad as a complete meal.

Prep time 20 minutes +
4 hours soaking
Cooking time 2½ hours
Serves 4–6

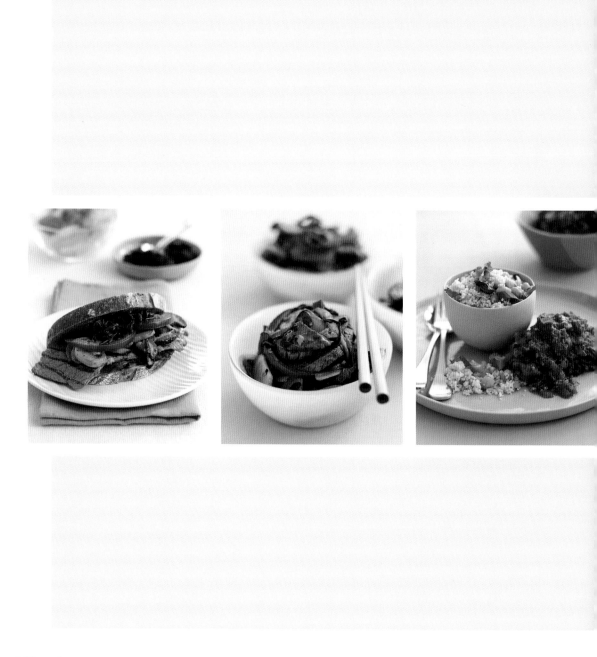

Main meals

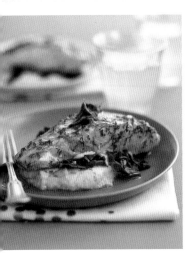 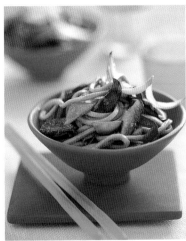 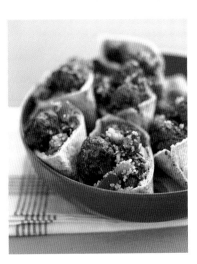

nutrition per serve   Energy **2686 kJ (642 Cal)** Fat **19.4 g** Saturated fat **8 g**
Protein **65.3 g** Carbohydrate **41.6 g** Fibre **6 g** Cholesterol **173 mg** Sodium **552 mg**

Lamb souvlaki

2 tsp olive oil

2 tsp finely grated lemon zest

80 ml (2½ fl oz/⅓ cup) lemon juice

2 tsp dried oregano

125 ml (4 fl oz/½ cup) dry white
   wine

3 garlic cloves, finely chopped

2 fresh bay leaves

1 kg (2 lb 4 oz) boned leg lamb

250 g (9 oz/1 cup) low-fat plain
   yoghurt

2 garlic cloves, crushed, extra

olive oil spray

4 wholemeal (whole-wheat) pitta
   breads, to serve

Prep time 20 minutes +
overnight marinating
Cooking time 10 minutes
Serves 4

1 To make the marinade, combine the oil, lemon zest,
lemon juice, oregano, wine, garlic and bay leaves in a
large non-metallic bowl. Season with salt (if desired)
and freshly ground black pepper. Trim the lamb and cut
into bite-sized cubes. Add to the marinade and toss to
coat well. Cover and refrigerate overnight.

2 Put the yoghurt and extra garlic in a bowl, mix together
well and leave for 30 minutes. If using wooden skewers,
soak them in cold water for about 30 minutes, to
prevent the skewers burning during cooking.

3 Drain lamb and pat dry. Thread lamb onto eight metal
or wooden skewers. Spray the barbecue hotplate with
oil and heat to high. Add lamb skewers and cook,
turning them often, for 7–8 minutes, or until evenly
brown on the outside and still a little rare in the middle.

4 Meanwhile, wrap the pitta breads in foil and put in
a warm place on the barbecue for 10 minutes to heat
through. Drizzle the lamb skewers with the garlic
yoghurt and serve on the warm pitta bread with a
green salad.

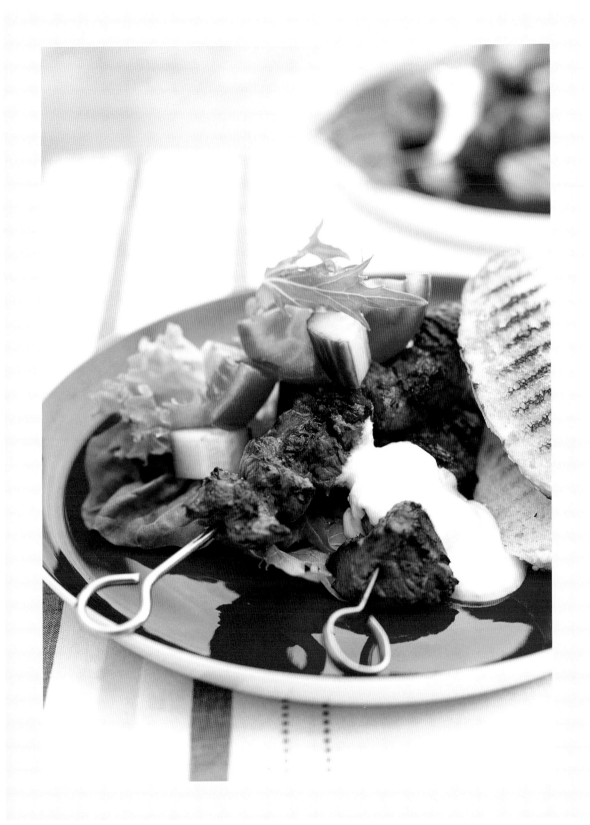

Moroccan chicken

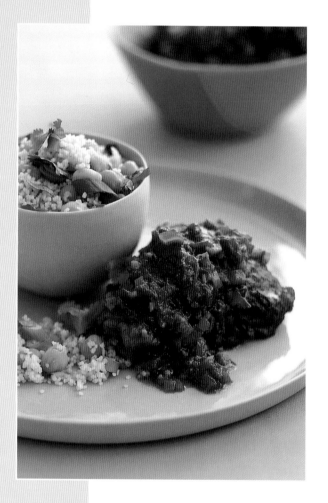

1 tsp cumin seeds
1 tsp coriander seeds
1 tsp ground ginger
1 tsp ground turmeric
1 tsp ground cinnamon
$\frac{1}{2}$ tsp chilli flakes
8 skinless chicken pieces
3 tsp olive oil
1 onion, finely chopped
3 garlic cloves, crushed
1 tsp finely grated fresh ginger
400 g (14 oz) tin chopped tomatoes
250 ml (9 fl oz/1 cup) chicken stock

nutrition per serve

Energy **2845 kJ (680 Cal)** Fat **17.5 g** Saturated fat **4.3 g** Protein **55.4 g** Carbohydrate **70.5 g** Fibre **6.5 g** Cholesterol **170 mg** Sodium **984 mg**

Couscous

375 ml (13 fl oz/1½ cups) chicken stock

1 garlic clove, crushed

280 g (10 oz/1½ cups) couscous

400 g (14 oz) tin chickpeas

3 spring onions (scallions), thinly sliced on the diagonal

3 tbsp chopped coriander (cilantro) leaves

Prep time 20 minutes + 15 minutes standing

Cooking time 1 hour

Serves 4

1 Put the cumin seeds, coriander seeds, ground ginger, turmeric, cinnamon and chilli flakes in a small heavy-based frying pan. Cook, stirring, over medium heat for 1 minute, or until fragrant. Grind the spices using a mortar and pestle or spice grinder to make a powder.

2 Sprinkle the chicken pieces with the spice mixture, rubbing in well. Heat 2 teaspoons of the oil in a large, deep heavy-based frying pan. Add the chicken and cook for 8 minutes, turning the pieces to brown evenly. Remove from the pan and set aside.

3 Add the remaining oil to the pan and cook the onion, garlic and ginger over medium heat for 3 minutes, or until softened. Add the tomatoes, stock and chicken to the pan. Bring to the boil, reduce the heat to low, cover and simmer for 45 minutes, or until the chicken is tender and the sauce has reduced. Season to taste.

4 Meanwhile, make the couscous. Put the stock and garlic in a small saucepan and bring to the boil. Put couscous in a bowl and pour over the hot stock. Cover with plastic wrap and set aside for 15 minutes. Stir couscous with a fork to fluff up the grains, then add rinsed and drained chickpeas, spring onion and half the coriander leaves. Season well. Serve the couscous with the Moroccan chicken. Sprinkle with the remaining coriander.

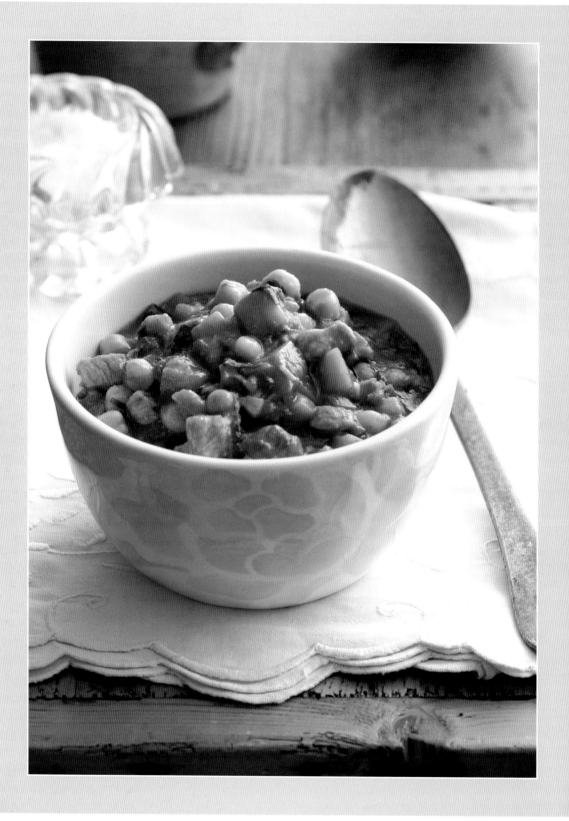

nutrition per serve   Energy **1128 kJ (269 Cal)** Fat **8.6 g** Saturated fat **1.7 g**
Protein **28.5 g** Carbohydrate **16.5 g** Fibre **6.5 g** Cholesterol **95 mg** Sodium **488 mg**

Pork and chickpea stew

2 tsp ground cumin

1 tsp ground coriander

½ tsp chilli powder

¼ tsp ground cinnamon

400 g (14 oz) lean diced pork,
    trimmed

1 tbsp plain (all-purpose) flour

1 tbsp olive oil

1 large onion, finely chopped

3 garlic cloves, finely chopped

2 large unpeeled carrots, chopped

2 celery stalks, sliced

250 ml (9 fl oz/1 cup) chicken stock

2 ripe tomatoes, chopped

310 g (11 oz) tin chickpeas, drained
    and rinsed

2 tbsp chopped parsley

1 Cook the spices in a dry frying pan over low heat, shaking the pan, for 1 minute, or until the spices are fragrant.

2 Combine the trimmed pork with the spices and flour in a plastic bag and toss well to coat. Remove the pork from the bag and shake off the excess flour.

3 Heat the oil in a large heavy-based saucepan over high heat and cook the pork, tossing regularly, for 8 minutes, or until lightly browned. Add the onion, garlic, carrot, celery and half the stock to the pan and toss well. Cover and cook for 10 minutes.

4 Add the remaining stock and tomato and season with salt and freshly ground black pepper. Bring to the boil, reduce the heat and cover with a tight-fitting lid, then simmer over low heat for 1 hour. Gently shake the pan occasionally but don't remove the lid during cooking. Stir in the chickpeas and parsley. Simmer, uncovered, for a further 5 minutes and serve.

Prep time 30 minutes
Cooking time 1½ hours
Serves 4

nutrition per serve Energy **2386 kJ (570 Cal)** Fat **8.1 g** Saturated fat **2.9 g**
Protein **45.3 g** Carbohydrate **75 g** Fibre **5 g** Cholesterol **99 mg** Sodium **386 mg**

Beef stroganoff

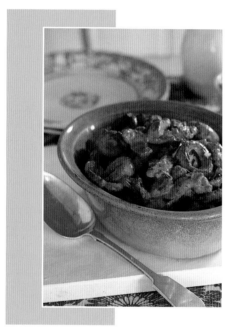

500 g (1 lb 2 oz) lean beef rump steak

olive oil spray

1 onion, sliced

¼ tsp paprika

250 g (9 oz) button mushrooms, halved

2 tbsp tomato paste (concentrated purée)

125 ml (4 fl oz/½ cup) beef stock

375 g (13 oz) fettucine

125 ml (4 fl oz/½ cup) evaporated skim milk

3 tsp cornflour (cornstarch)

3 tbsp chopped parsley

Prep time 20 minutes

Cooking time 30 minutes

Serves 4

1 Trim the beef and slice it into thin strips. Heat a large non-stick frying pan over high heat and spray with the oil. Add the beef in batches and cook for 2–3 minutes, or until just cooked. Remove from the pan.

2 Lightly spray the pan with oil again and cook the onion, paprika and mushrooms over medium heat until the onion has softened. Add the beef, tomato paste, stock and 125 ml (4 fl oz/½ cup) water. Bring to the boil, then reduce the heat and simmer for 10 minutes.

3 Meanwhile, cook the pasta in a large saucepan of boiling water for 10 minutes, or until al dente. Drain well.

4 Mix the evaporated milk with the cornflour in a small bowl. Add to the pan and stir until the sauce boils and thickens. Sprinkle with parsley and serve with the fettucine. Serve with a salad or steamed vegetables.

nutrition per serve Energy **1611 kJ (385 Cal)** Fat **6.8 g** Saturated fat **1.4 g**
Protein **35.3 g** Carbohydrate **42.1 g** Fibre **5.3 g** Cholesterol **87 mg** Sodium **809 mg**

Chicken and noodle stir-fry

200 g (7 oz) dried rice noodles

3 tbsp chopped fresh ginger

2 garlic cloves, finely chopped

1 tsp sesame oil

**200 g (7 oz) broccolini, cut into
5 cm (2 in) pieces**

**1 large red capsicum (pepper),
thinly sliced**

**100 g (3½ oz) snowpeas (mangetout)
or sugar snap peas, thinly sliced
on the diagonal**

4 spring onions (scallions), sliced

2 tsp olive oil

**500 g (1 lb 2 oz) boneless skinless
chicken breasts, cut into strips**

1 tbsp black bean sauce

1 tbsp oyster sauce or soy sauce

1 tbsp hoisin sauce

**1 tbsp chilli sauce or ½ large chilli,
finely chopped**

**80 ml (2½ fl oz/⅓ cup) chicken stock
or water**

**4 tbsp roughly chopped coriander
(cilantro) leaves and stalks**

1 Soak the rice noodles in hot water, immersing them completely. Mix well to break up the noodles and prevent them sticking together. Leave to soften for 10 minutes, then drain.

2 Meanwhile, put the ginger and garlic in a wok. Pour the sesame oil over the top and turn the heat to high. Cook for about 1 minute, or until the wok is hot. Add the vegetables and cook for 2 minutes, stirring frequently, until tender. Transfer the vegetables to a bowl.

3 Heat the olive oil in the wok, add the chicken strips and stir-fry for 2 minutes, or until just cooked. Add the black bean sauce, oyster sauce, hoisin sauce and chilli sauce. Stir to combine, then transfer the chicken to the bowl with the vegetables, leaving behind as much liquid as possible in the wok.

4 Add the drained noodles and stock to the wok and cook for 1–2 minutes, or until the noodles are soft. Return the chicken and vegetables to the wok along with the coriander. Remove from the heat and stir until well mixed. Serve immediately.

Prep time 20 minutes + 10 minutes soaking
Cooking time 10 minutes
Serves 4

nutrition per serve   Energy 1727 kJ (413 Cal) Fat 11 g Saturated fat 3.1 g
Protein 27.7 g Carbohydrate 47.6 g Fibre 6.8 g Cholesterol 59 mg Sodium 2012 mg

Beef and hokkien noodle stir-fry

600 g (1 lb 5 oz) fresh hokkien
   (egg) noodles

olive oil spray

350 g (12 oz) lean beef fillet, partially
   frozen, thinly sliced

1 tbsp peanut oil

1 large onion, cut into thin wedges

1 large carrot, thinly sliced on the
   diagonal

1 red capsicum (pepper), cut into
   thin strips

2 garlic cloves, crushed

1 tsp grated fresh ginger

100 g (3½ oz) snow peas
   (mangetout), sliced in half
   on the diagonal

200 g (7 oz) shiitake mushrooms,
   sliced

3 tbsp oyster sauce

2 tbsp light soy sauce

1 tbsp soft brown sugar

½ tsp five-spice powder

1 Put the noodles in a heatproof bowl with enough
   boiling water to cover. Leave to soften for 1 minute,
   separate noodles with a fork, then drain and set aside.

2 Spray a large wok with oil and heat over high heat.
   Add the beef in batches and cook until brown.
   Remove and keep warm.

3 Heat the peanut oil in the wok, and when very hot,
   add the onion, carrot and capsicum and stir-fry for
   2–3 minutes, or until tender. Add the garlic, ginger,
   snow peas and shiitake mushrooms and cook for
   another minute, then return the beef to the wok.

4 Add the noodles to the wok, tossing well. Combine the
   oyster sauce with the soy sauce, sugar, five-spice powder
   and 1 tablespoon water and pour over the noodles. Toss
   until warmed through and serve immediately.

Prep time 15 minutes
Cooking time 15 minutes
Serves 4

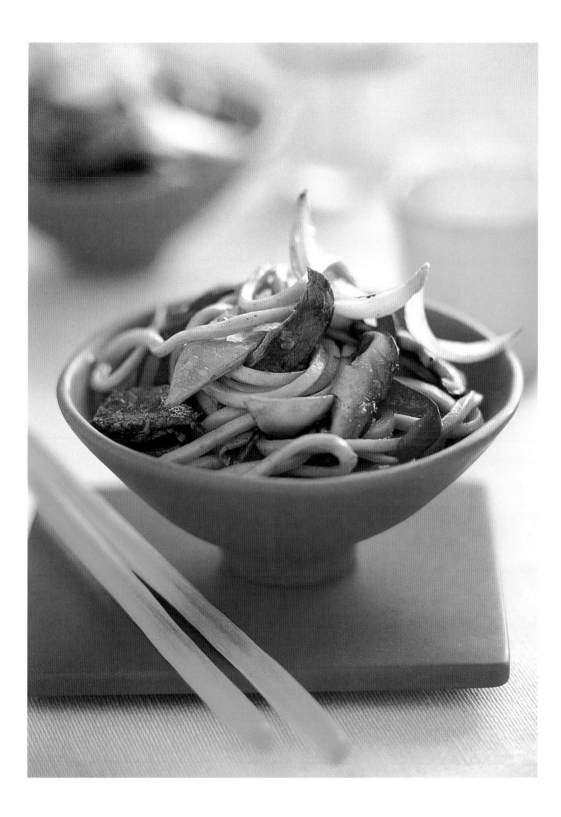

nutrition per serve (6)   Energy **2369 kJ (566 Cal)** Fat **17.7 g** Saturated fat **5.5 g** Protein **39.2 g** Carbohydrate **56.9 g** Fibre **9.3 g** Cholesterol **111 mg** Sodium **509 mg**

Chicken and zucchini stew

2 tsp olive oil

8 boneless skinless chicken thighs, trimmed

1 onion, thinly sliced

4 garlic cloves, finely chopped

3 tbsp white wine

250 ml (9 fl oz/1 cup) chicken stock

1 tbsp finely chopped rosemary

1 tsp grated lemon zest

1 bay leaf

2 x 400 g (14 oz) tins cannellini beans, drained and rinsed

3 zucchini (courgettes), halved lengthways, then sliced on the diagonal

375 g (13 oz) fusilli

Prep time 20 minutes

Cooking time 1 hour 10 minutes

Serves 4–6

1   Heat the oil in a large flameproof casserole dish. Add the chicken in batches and cook over medium heat for 4 minutes on each side, or until browned. Remove the chicken from the dish. Add the onion and cook for 5 minutes, or until softened. Add the garlic and cook for 1 minute, or until fragrant, then pour in the wine and stock and bring to the boil, scraping the bottom of the dish to remove any sediment.

2   Return the chicken and any juices to the dish along with the rosemary, lemon zest and bay leaf. Reduce the heat to low and simmer, covered, for 40 minutes, or until the chicken is tender. Stir in the cannellini beans and zucchini and cook for a further 5 minutes, or until the zucchini is tender.

3   Meanwhile, cook the pasta in a large saucepan of boiling water for 10 minutes, or until al dente. Drain and serve with the chicken. Serve with a mixed leaf salad dressed with oil and vinegar.

nutrition per serve
Energy **2418 kJ (578 Cal)** Fat **12.2 g** Saturated fat **4.1 g**
Protein **36.3 g** Carbohydrate **75.5 g** Fibre **7.8 g** Cholesterol **64 mg** Sodium **405 mg**

Chilli con carne with parsley rice

2 tsp olive oil

1 onion, chopped

3 garlic cloves, crushed

1 celery stalk, sliced

500 g (1 lb 2 oz) lean minced
   (ground) beef

2 tsp chilli powder

pinch of cayenne pepper

1 tbsp chopped oregano

400 g (14 oz) tin chopped tomatoes

2 tbsp tomato paste (concentrated
   purée)

300 g (10½ oz/1½ cups) basmati
   rice, rinsed and drained

4 tbsp finely chopped parsley

1 tsp soft brown sugar

1 tbsp cider vinegar or red wine
   vinegar

400 g (14 oz) tin red kidney beans,
   drained and rinsed

plain yoghurt or grated low-fat
   cheddar cheese, to serve

1 Heat the oil in a large heavy-based saucepan. Add the onion, garlic and celery and stir over medium heat for 5 minutes, or until softened. Add the beef and cook over high heat for 5 minutes, or until well browned. Add the chilli powder, cayenne pepper and oregano. Stir well and cook for a further 5 minutes.

2 Add the tomatoes, tomato paste and 125 ml (4 fl oz/ ½ cup) water, stir well, then simmer for 30 minutes, stirring occasionally.

3 Meanwhile, put the rice and 750 ml (26 fl oz/3 cups) water in a saucepan and bring to the boil over medium heat. Reduce the heat to low, cover and cook for 20 minutes, or until the rice is tender. Remove from the heat and leave to stand, covered, for 5 minutes.

4 Add the parsley, sugar, vinegar and beans to the chilli mixture and season with salt (if desired) and freshly ground black pepper. Heat through for 5 minutes before serving. Serve with the rice and top with a little yoghurt or cheese, if you like.

Prep time 15 minutes
Cooking time 1 hour 10 minutes
Serves 4

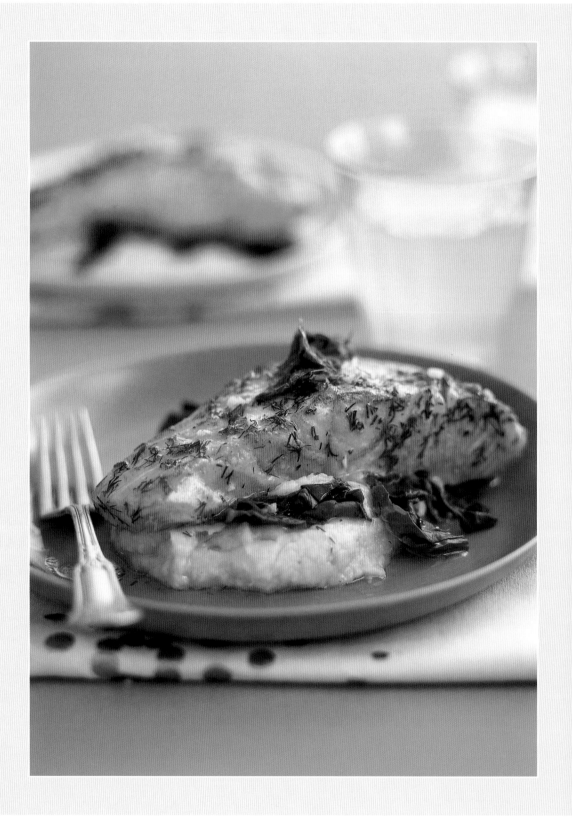

nutrition per serve   Energy **1710 kJ (409 Cal)** Fat **15.9 g** Saturated fat **3.2 mg**
Protein **47.1 g** Carbohydrate **15.1 g** Fibre **10.2 g** Cholesterol **95 mg** Sodium **563 mg**

Salmon with bean puree

4 x 180 g (6 oz) salmon fillets

2 tsp canola oil

1 garlic clove, crushed

2 tbsp white wine vinegar

1 tsp finely grated lime zest

2 tbsp chopped dill

600 g (1 lb 5 oz) tinned cannellini
   beans, drained and rinsed,
   to yield about 380 g (13½ oz)
   drained beans

1 bay leaf

250 ml (9 fl oz/1 cup) chicken stock

500 g (1 lb 2 oz/1 bunch) baby
   English spinach leaves, roughly
   chopped

Prep time 15 minutes +
10 minutes marinating

Cooking time 25 minutes

Serves 4

1 Put the salmon in a non-metallic dish. Combine the oil, garlic, vinegar, lime zest and dill, pour over the fish, then cover and leave to marinate for 10 minutes.

2 Put the beans, bay leaf and stock in a saucepan, bring to the boil, then reduce the heat and simmer for 10 minutes. Remove the bay leaf. Cool a little, then transfer to a food processor and purée. Season well with salt (if desired) and freshly ground black pepper.

3 Drain the salmon, reserving the marinade. Heat a non-stick frying pan over high heat, add the salmon and cook for 3–5 minutes on each side, or until crisp and golden. Remove from the pan and set aside. Add the marinade to the pan and bring to the boil.

4 Steam the spinach until wilted. Place a mound of bean purée on each serving plate and top with the wilted spinach and salmon fillets. Drizzle over the marinade. Serve with chunky slices of brown bread and a side dish of steamed squash or sweet corn.

Spaghetti with meatballs

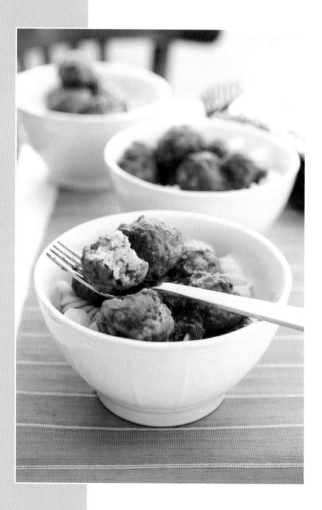

500 g (1 lb 2 oz) lean minced (ground) beef

40 g (1½ oz/½ cup) fresh wholegrain breadcrumbs

1 small onion, finely chopped

2 garlic cloves, crushed

2 tsp worcestershire sauce

1 tsp dried oregano

30 g (1 oz/¼ cup) plain (all-purpose) flour

1 tbsp olive oil

400 g (14 oz) spaghetti

nutrition per serve
Energy **2899 kJ (693 Cal)** Fat **16.4 g** Saturated fat **4.7 g**
Protein **41.6 g** Carbohydrate **89.1 g** Fibre **8.2 g** Cholesterol **64 mg** Sodium **520 mg**

Sauce

2 x 400 g (14 oz) tins chopped
   tomatoes

1 tsp olive oil

1 onion, finely chopped

2 garlic cloves, crushed

2 tbsp tomato paste (concentrated
   purée)

125 ml (4 fl oz/½ cup) beef stock

Prep time 30 minutes

Cooking time 40 minutes

Serves 4

1 To make the meatballs, combine the beef, breadcrumbs, onion, garlic, worcestershire sauce and oregano in a bowl. Season with salt (if desired) and freshly ground black pepper. Use your hands to mix the ingredients together. Roll level tablespoons of the mixture into balls, dust lightly with the flour and shake off the excess.

2 Heat the oil in a deep frying pan and cook the meatballs in batches, turning frequently, until browned all over. Drain well on paper towels. Wipe the pan out with paper towels.

3 To make the sauce, purée the tomatoes in a food processor or blender. Heat the oil in the frying pan, add the onion and cook over medium heat for 2–3 minutes, or until soft and lightly golden. Add the garlic and cook for a further 1 minute. Add the puréed tomatoes, tomato paste and stock to the pan and stir to combine. Bring mixture to the boil, then add meatballs. Reduce heat and simmer for 15 minutes, turning meatballs once. Season with freshly ground black pepper.

4 Meanwhile, cook the spaghetti in a large saucepan of boiling water for 10 minutes, or until al dente. Drain well, then divide among four plates and top with the meatballs and sauce. Serve with a mixed green salad.

Pork and black bean stir-fry

300 g (10½ oz/1½ cups) brown
  basmati rice, rinsed and drained

400 g (14 oz) lean pork leg steaks

2 tsp sesame oil

2 onions, thinly sliced

2 garlic cloves, finely chopped

2–3 tsp chopped fresh ginger

1 red capsicum (pepper), cut into
  strips

1 tbsp salted black beans, rinsed,
  roughly chopped

500 g (1 lb 2 oz) baby bok choy
  (pak choy), shredded

80 g (2¾ oz/½ cup) drained and
  rinsed tinned water chestnuts,
  thinly sliced

2 tbsp oyster sauce

1 tbsp soy sauce

2 tsp fish sauce

Prep time 20 minutes

Cooking time 1 hour

Serves 4

1 Put 1.5 litres (52 fl oz/6 cups) water in a saucepan and
bring to the boil over medium heat. Add the rice and
cook for 30–35 minutes, stirring occasionally, until the
rice is tender.

2 Meanwhile, slice the pork into strips across the grain.
Heat a wok over medium–high heat, then add half the
sesame oil and swirl to coat the wok. Add the onion,
garlic and ginger to the wok and cook for 3–4 minutes,
being careful that the garlic doesn't burn. Then add the
capsicum and cook for 2–3 minutes. Remove from the
wok.

3 Heat the remaining sesame oil in the wok, add the pork
in batches and briefly stir-fry until browned. Reheat the
wok between batches.

4 Return all the pork to the wok along with the capsicum
mixture, black beans, bok choy and water chestnuts.
Stir in the oyster sauce, soy sauce and fish sauce. Toss
quickly, reduce the heat, then cover and steam for
3–4 minutes, or until the bok choy has just wilted.
Serve the stir-fry with the brown rice.

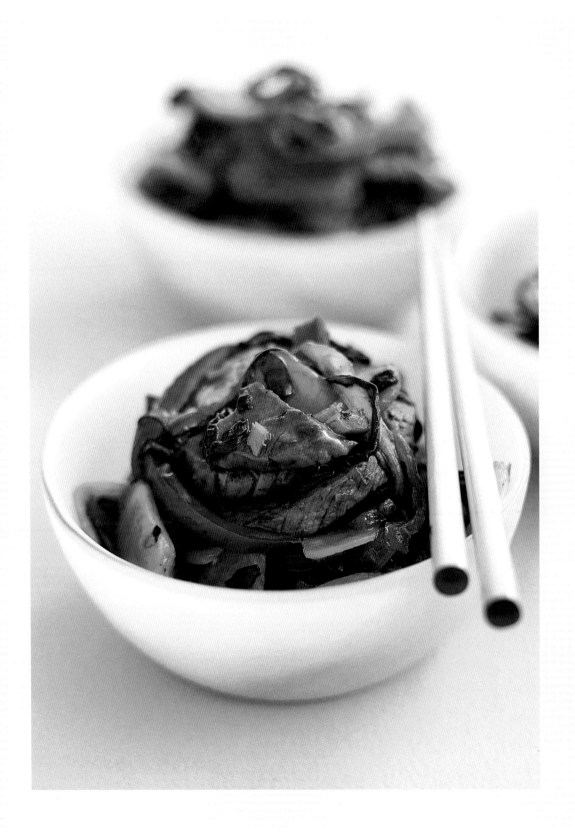

Lamb stir-fry

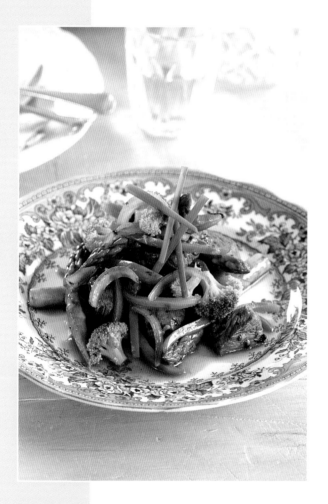

2 tsp green peppercorns, finely chopped

3 garlic cloves, finely chopped

1 tbsp canola oil

400 g (14 oz) lean lamb fillets, trimmed

300 g (10½ oz/1½ cups) brown basmati rice, rinsed and drained

canola oil spray

1 onion, cut into small wedges

80 ml (2½ fl oz/⅓ cup) dry sherry

1 green capsicum (pepper), cut into strips

20 small asparagus spears, trimmed and cut into bite-sized pieces

nutrition per serve
Energy **2241 kJ (535 Cal)** Fat **11.8 g** Saturated fat **2.5 g** Protein **33.1 g** Carbohydrate **64.9 g** Fibre **7.5 g** Cholesterol **65 mg** Sodium **574 mg**

250 g (9 oz) broccoli florets

50 g (1¾ oz/⅓ cup) tinned or frozen soya beans

2 tbsp oyster sauce

garlic chives, snipped into short lengths, to garnish

Prep time 20 minutes + 20 minutes marinating

Cooking time 55 minutes

Serves 4

1   To make the marinade, put the green peppercorns, garlic and oil in a large bowl. Add the trimmed lamb and toss well to coat. Cover with plastic wrap and marinate for 20 minutes.

2   Put 1.5 litres (52 fl oz/6 cups) water in a saucepan and bring to the boil over medium heat. Add the rice and cook for 30–35 minutes, stirring occasionally, until the rice is tender.

3   Remove the lamb from the marinade and cut into bite-sized pieces. Spray a wok with oil and heat over high heat until slightly smoking. Add the lamb in small batches and stir-fry briefly until browned and just cooked. Remove from the wok and keep warm. Reheat the wok between batches.

4   Reheat the wok, spray with oil and stir-fry the onion and 2 teaspoons of the sherry for 1 minute. Add the capsicum and a large pinch of salt (if desired). Cover, steam for 2 minutes, then add the asparagus, broccoli and the remaining sherry and stir-fry for 1 minute. Cover and steam for 3 minutes, or until the vegetables are just tender. Return the lamb to the wok along with the soya beans to heat through, add the oyster sauce and stir to combine with the vegetables. Garnish with the chives and serve with the brown rice.

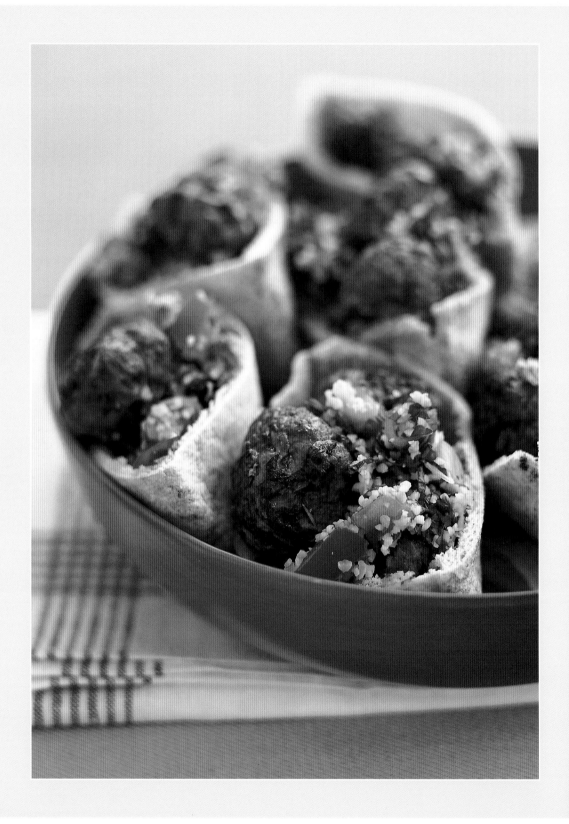

nutrition per serve   Energy **2200 kJ (525 Cal)** Fat **8.1 g** Saturated fat **2.6 g**
Protein **40.5 g** Carbohydrate **63.9 g** Fibre **12 g** Cholesterol **84 mg** Sodium **753 mg**

Lamb koftas in pitta bread

500 g (1 lb 2 oz) lean lamb

1 onion, roughly chopped

1 large handful flat-leaf (Italian) parsley, roughly chopped

1 large handful mint, roughly chopped

2 tsp lemon zest

1 tsp ground cumin

¼ tsp chilli powder

250 g (9 oz/1 cup) low-fat plain yoghurt

2 tsp lemon juice

olive oil spray

4 wholemeal (whole-wheat) pitta breads

Tabouleh

90 g (3¼ oz/½ cup) burghul (bulgur)

2 vine-ripened tomatoes

1 Lebanese (short) cucumber

60 g (2¼ oz/½ bunch) flat-leaf (Italian) parsley, chopped

1 large handful mint, chopped

2 French shallots, chopped

125 ml (4 fl oz/½ cup) fat-free Greek or Italian dressing

1 Roughly chop the lamb. Put lamb and onion in a food processor and process until smooth. Add parsley, mint, lemon zest and spices and process until well combined. Divide mixture into 24 balls and place on a tray. Cover and refrigerate for 30 minutes for the flavours to develop.

2 Meanwhile, to make the tabouleh, put burghul in a bowl. Cover with boiling water, set aside for 10 minutes, or until softened. Drain, then use clean hands to squeeze dry. Cut tomatoes in half, scoop out the seeds with a teaspoon, then chop the flesh. Cut cucumber in halves lengthways, scoop out the seeds, then chop the flesh. Put the burghul, tomato and cucumber in a large bowl with the parsley, mint and shallots. Stir in the dressing.

3 To make the yoghurt dressing, combine the yoghurt and lemon juice in a bowl. Cover and refrigerate until needed.

4 Heat a large, non-stick frying pan over medium heat and spray with the oil. Cook the lamb balls in two batches, spraying the pan with oil before each batch, until browned all over and cooked through.

5 Preheat the oven to 180°C (350°F/Gas 4). Cut the pitta breads in half, wrap in foil and place in the oven for 10 minutes to warm. To serve, divide the tabouleh among the pitta bread halves, add three kofta balls to each and top with the yoghurt dressing.

Prep time 35 minutes + 30 minutes resting
Cooking time 15 minutes
Serves 4

nutrition per serve   Energy **1598 kJ (382 Cal)** Fat **11.8 g** Saturated fat **4.2 g**
Protein **50.9 g** Carbohydrate **11.2 g** Fibre **8.2 g** Cholesterol **63 mg** Sodium **1504 mg**

Seared tuna with sesame greens

80 ml (2½ fl oz/⅓ cup) soy sauce

3 tbsp mirin

1 tbsp sake

1 tsp caster (superfine) sugar

1 tsp finely grated fresh ginger

2 tsp lemon juice

4 x 175 g (6 oz) tuna steaks

olive oil spray

350 g (12 oz/1 bunch) choy sum
    (Chinese flowering cabbage),
    trimmed and halved

800 g (1 lb 12 oz/1 bunch) Chinese
    broccoli (gai larn), trimmed and
    halved

2 tsp sesame seeds, lightly toasted

1 Combine the soy sauce, mirin, sake, sugar, ginger and lemon juice together in a bowl, stirring to dissolve the sugar. Put the tuna in a shallow non-metallic dish and spoon the soy marinade over the top. Turn the tuna in the marinade so it is well coated. Cover and leave to marinate in the refrigerator for 30 minutes.

2 Preheat a chargrill pan over high heat and spray with oil. Lift tuna out of the marinade, reserving the marinade. Cook tuna for 1½–2 minutes on each side, until cooked on the outside but still pink in the middle.

3 Pour the marinade into a large frying pan. Bring the liquid to the boil, add the choy sum, Chinese broccoli and sesame seeds to the simmering sauce. Cook, turning vegetables until lightly wilted, then place onto serving plates. Top the vegetables with tuna and spoon marinade over the top. Serve with rice or noodles.

Prep time 15 minutes +
30 minutes marinating
Cooking time 10 minutes
Serves 4

nutrition per serve Energy **2483 kJ (593 Cal)** Fat **27 g** Saturated fat **7.5 g**
Protein **42.9 g** Carbohydrate **39.9 g** Fibre **8.4 g** Cholesterol **178 mg** Sodium **165 mg**

Lemon chicken with vegetables

1.4 kg (3 lb 2 oz) chicken

2 bay leaves

2 lemons

2 lemon thyme sprigs

2 marjoram sprigs

1 tbsp chopped lemon thyme

1 tbsp chopped marjoram

1 tbsp olive oil

12 baby new potatoes, unpeeled

300 g (10½ oz) orange sweet potato, peeled and cut into 8 pieces

8 French shallots, unpeeled

2 large zucchini (courgettes), halved lengthways, then halved again widthways

8 garlic cloves, unpeeled

Prep time 20 minutes

Cooking time 1 hour 10 minutes + 5 minutes resting

Serves 4

1 Preheat the oven to 200°C (400°F/Gas 6). Pat the chicken dry with paper towels and place on a rack in a deep roasting tin. Season the cavity and put the bay leaves, 1 whole lemon and the lemon thyme and marjoram sprigs inside. Cut the remaining lemon in half and rub all over the chicken, then cut the lemon into quarters and reserve.

2 Season lightly and roast the chicken, basting every 20 minutes with the tin juices, for 1 hour 10 minutes, or until browned and the juices run clear when pierced between the thigh and the body. Remove the chicken from the rack and sit, covered lightly with foil, for 5 minutes.

3 Meanwhile, to roast the vegetables, combine the chopped lemon thyme and marjoram with the oil, salt (if desired), freshly ground black pepper and the reserved lemon quarters in a large bowl. Add all the vegetables and the unpeeled garlic cloves and toss together.

4 Put the potatoes, sweet potato and French shallots in a single layer in a large roasting tin. Place in the oven 20 minutes after chicken and roast for 25 minutes, then add zucchini, cut side down, and garlic cloves. Cook for a further 25 minutes, or until golden and tender, turning the vegetables occasionally to ensure they don't burn. Discard the lemon and serve the chicken with the roast vegetables and peeled garlic cloves.

Steak sandwich with onion relish

Red onion relish

1 tsp olive oil

2 red onions, thinly sliced

2 tbsp soft brown sugar

2 tbsp balsamic vinegar

1 tbsp thyme

2 tsp olive oil

250 g (9 oz) mixed mushrooms
(flat, button, shiitake), sliced

olive oil spray

4 x 60 g (2¼ oz) lean minute beef
steaks, trimmed

125 g (4½ oz) baby English spinach
leaves

8 slices wholegrain bread

1 large tomato, sliced

Prep time 20 minutes

Cooking time 25 minutes

Serves 4

1 To make the red onion relish, heat the oil in a saucepan, add the onion and cook over low heat for 10 minutes, or until softened, stirring frequently and taking care not to burn. Add the sugar and balsamic vinegar and cook, stirring, for 10–12 minutes, or until softened and slightly syrupy. Stir in the thyme.

2 Meanwhile, heat the olive oil in a heavy-based frying pan over medium heat. Stir in the mushrooms, then add 2 tablespoons water. Cover, then reduce heat and simmer for 5 minutes, or until softened, making sure the mushrooms don't dry out. Stir once or twice. Remove lid and increase heat to allow any juice to evaporate. Season with freshly ground black pepper.

3 Lightly spray a chargrill pan or frying pan with oil. Add the steak and cook for 1 minute on each side, or until cooked to your liking. Very briefly microwave or steam the spinach until just wilted. Drain away any juices.

4 Toast the bread and arrange one slice of toast on each plate. Top with the spinach, then the steak, mushrooms and tomato and finish with a dollop of the onion relish. Top with the remaining slice of toast. Serve with a mixed green salad.

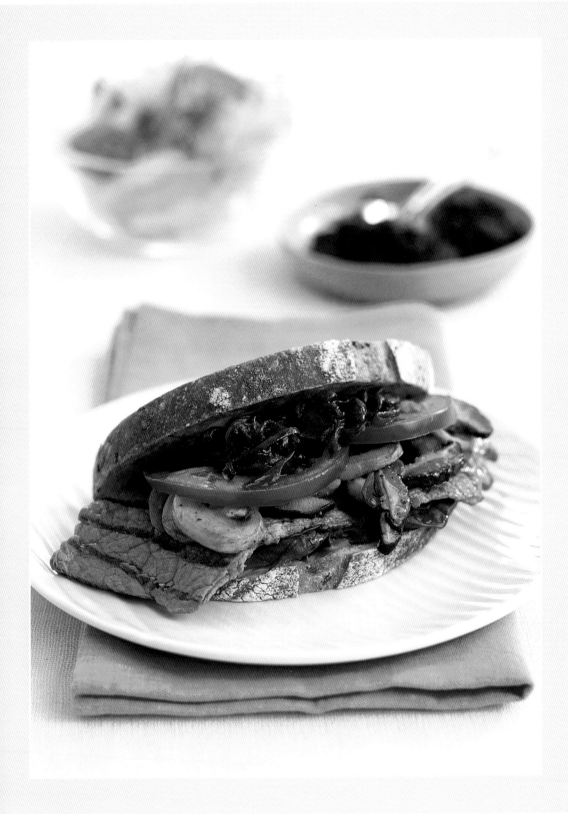

Beef and vegetable curry

2 tsp olive oil

1 large onion, chopped

2 garlic cloves, crushed

1 tbsp grated fresh ginger

2 tsp chopped red chilli

2 tsp ground cumin

2 tsp ground coriander

1 tsp ground cardamom

1 tsp ground turmeric

½ tsp ground cloves

750 g (1 lb 10 oz) lean beef, such as
   chuck or blade, cubed

400 g (14 oz) tin crushed tomatoes

250 ml (9 fl oz/1 cup) beef stock

650 g (1 lb 7 oz) unpeeled potatoes,
   cut into large chunks

125 g (4½ oz) green beans, sliced

2 carrots, sliced

125 g (4½ oz/½ cup) low-fat plain
   yoghurt

1 Heat the oil in a large pan, add the onion and cook
over low heat for 15 minutes, stirring regularly, until
soft. Add the garlic, ginger, chilli and spices and stir
for 1 minute.

2 Add the beef and stir to coat with the spices. Add the
tomatoes and beef stock and bring to the boil. Reduce
the heat to very low, cover and simmer for 1½ hours.

3 Add the potato and cook for a further 25 minutes,
then uncover, add the beans and carrots and cook for
15 minutes, or until the vegetables are tender and the
sauce thickens. Stir in the yoghurt, heat through and
serve with white or brown basmati rice.

Prep time 30 minutes

Cooking time 2½ hours

Serves 4

Energy **1874 kJ (448 Cal)** Fat **9.8 g** Saturated fat **3.8 g**
Protein **35.4 g** Carbohydrate **49.7 g** Fibre **7 g** Cholesterol **65 mg** Sodium **557 mg**

Shepherd's pie

olive oil spray

2 onions, thinly sliced

1 large carrot, finely chopped

2 celery stalks, finely chopped

500 g (1 lb 2 oz) lean minced
(ground) lamb

2 tbsp plain (all-purpose) flour

2 tbsp tomato paste (concentrated
purée)

2 tbsp worcestershire sauce

1 beef or chicken stock cube

1.25 kg (2 lb 12 oz) potatoes, peeled
and chopped

125 ml (4 fl oz/½ cup) skim milk

2 large handfuls parsley, finely
chopped

paprika, to sprinkle

Prep time 20 minutes
Cooking time 50 minutes
Serves 4

1 Lightly spray a large non-stick frying pan with oil and
heat over medium heat. Add the onion, carrot and
celery and cook, stirring constantly, for 5 minutes, or
until the vegetables begin to soften. Add 1 tablespoon
water to prevent sticking. Remove from the pan and set
aside. Spray the pan with a little more oil, add the lamb
and cook, stirring, over high heat until well browned.

2 Add the flour and stir for 2–3 minutes. Return the
vegetables to the pan along with the tomato paste,
worcestershire sauce, stock cube and 500 ml (17 fl oz/
2 cups) water. Slowly bring to the boil. Reduce the heat,
cover and simmer for 20 minutes, stirring occasionally.

3 Meanwhile, steam or microwave the potato until tender.
Drain and mash until smooth. Add the milk, season
with salt (if desired) and freshly ground black pepper
and beat well.

4 Stir the parsley through the lamb and season. Preheat
a grill (broiler). Pour the lamb into a 1.5 litre (52 fl oz/
6 cup) heatproof dish. Spoon the mashed potato over
the top and spread it evenly with the back of the spoon.
Use a fork to roughen up the potato. Sprinkle with
paprika and grill (broil) until the potato is golden,
watching carefully because the potato browns quickly.
Serve with a green salad.

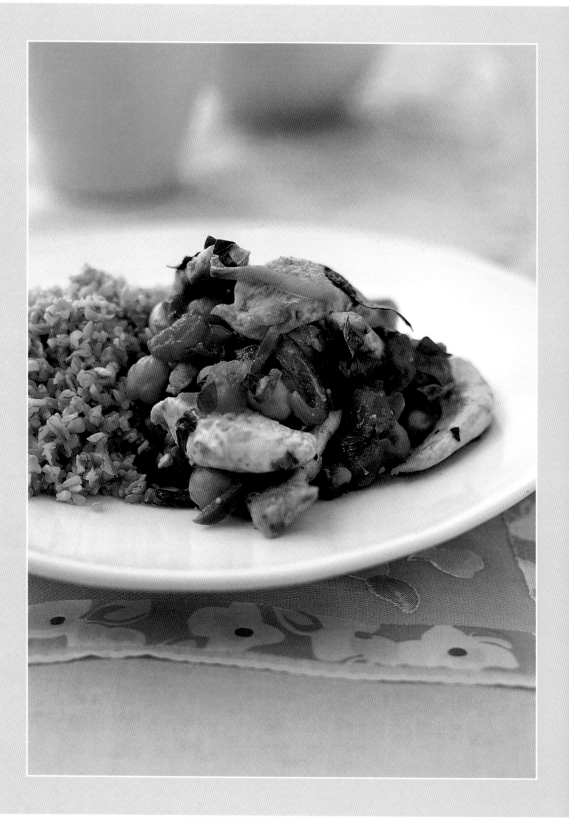

Middle-Eastern chicken

350 g (12 oz/2 cups) burghul
   (bulgur)

2 boneless skinless chicken breasts

2 tsp olive oil

1 red onion, thinly sliced

300 g (10½ oz) tin chickpeas,
   drained and rinsed

70 g (2½ oz/½ cup) unsalted
   pistachio kernels

1 tomato, chopped

juice of 1 orange

4 tbsp finely chopped flat-leaf
   (Italian) parsley

Prep time 15 minutes +
15 minutes soaking
Cooking time 20 minutes
Serves 4

1 Put the burghul in a bowl, cover with water and leave to soak for 15 minutes, or until the burghul has softened. Drain and use clean hands to squeeze dry.

2 Meanwhile, trim the chicken and thinly slice. Heat a large frying pan over high heat, add half the oil and swirl to coat. Add the chicken in batches and stir-fry for 3–5 minutes, or until cooked. Remove from the pan and keep warm. Reheat the pan between batches.

3 Add the remaining oil to the pan and cook the onion, stirring, for 2 minutes, then add the chickpeas, pistachios and tomato. Cook, stirring, for 3–5 minutes, or until the chickpeas are warmed through.

4 Pour in the orange juice, return the chicken and its juices to the pan and cook until half the juice has evaporated. Stir in the parsley. Season well with salt (if desired) and freshly ground black pepper and serve with the burghul.

nutrition per serve

Energy **2790 kJ (664 Cal)** Fat **10 g** Saturated fat **3.9 g**
Protein **39.5 g** Carbohydrate **97.5 g** Fibre **7.9 g** Cholesterol **154 mg** Sodium **799 mg**

Spaghetti marinara

125 g (4½ oz) small squid hoods

125 g (4½ oz) skinless firm white
    fish fillets

200 g (7 oz) raw prawns (shrimp)

12 mussels

2 tsp olive oil

1 onion, chopped

2 garlic cloves, crushed

125 ml (4 fl oz/½ cup) red wine

2 tbsp tomato paste (concentrated
    purée)

400 g (14 oz) tin chopped tomatoes

250 ml (9 fl oz/1 cup) bottled tomato
    pasta sauce

1 tbsp chopped basil

1 tbsp chopped oregano

20 g (¾ oz) canola margarine

500 g (1 lb 2 oz) spaghetti

Prep time 50 minutes
Cooking time 30 minutes
Serves 4

1 To prepare the seafood, slice the squid hoods into rings.
   Cut the fish into bite-sized cubes, checking for bones.
   Peel the prawns, leaving the tails intact. Gently pull out
   the dark vein from each prawn back, starting at the
   head end. Scrub the mussels with a stiff brush and pull
   out the hairy beards. Discard any mussels that are
   broken or any open ones that don't close when tapped
   on the bench.

2 Heat the olive oil in a large saucepan. Add the onion
   and garlic and cook over low heat for 2–3 minutes.
   Increase the heat to medium and add the wine, tomato
   paste, tomatoes and pasta sauce. Simmer, stirring
   occasionally, for 5–10 minutes, or until the sauce
   reduces and thickens slightly. Stir in the herbs and
   season to taste. Keep warm.

3 While the sauce is simmering, heat 125 ml (4 fl oz/
   ½ cup) water in a saucepan. Add the mussels, cover
   and steam for 3–5 minutes, or until the mussels have
   opened. Remove the mussels from the pan, discarding
   any that haven't opened, and stir the liquid left in the
   pan into the tomato sauce.

4 Heat the margarine in a frying pan and sauté the squid,
   fish and prawns in batches for 1–2 minutes, or until
   cooked. Add the seafood to the warm tomato sauce and
   stir gently.

5 Meanwhile, cook the pasta in a large saucepan of
   boiling water for 10 minutes, or until al dente. Drain
   and toss with the seafood sauce. Serve immediately
   with a green salad.

nutrition per serve (6) Energy **1866 kJ (446 Cal)** Fat **6.7 g** Saturated fat **1.7 g** Protein **19.8 g** Carbohydrate **72.8 g** Fibre **7.7 g** Cholesterol **23 mg** Sodium **506 mg**

Rigatoni and sausage

2 tsp olive oil

1 large onion, chopped

2 garlic cloves, crushed

4 lean beef sausages

2 x 400 g (14 oz) tins chopped
    tomatoes

400 g (14 oz) tin red kidney
    beans, drained and rinsed

2 tbsp chopped basil

1 tbsp chopped sage

1 tbsp chopped parsley

500 g (1 lb 2 oz) rigatoni

grated parmesan cheese,
    sto serve (optional)

1 Heat the oil in a large saucepan over medium heat. Add the onion, garlic and sausages and cook, stirring occasionally, for 5 minutes. Remove the sausages, chop them and return to the saucepan.

2 Add the tomatoes, kidney beans, basil, sage and parsley and season well with salt (if desired) and freshly ground black pepper. Reduce the heat and simmer for 20 minutes.

3 Meanwhile, cook the pasta in a large saucepan of boiling water for 10 minutes, or until al dente. Drain well. Divide among bowls and top with the sauce. If you like, sprinkle with parmesan before serving.

Prep time 25 minutes

Cooking time 35 minutes

Serves 4–6

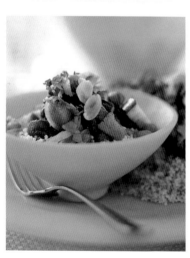
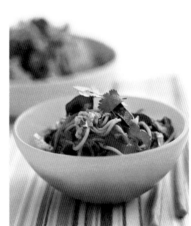
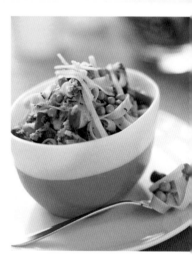

Vegetarian meals

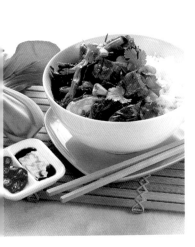 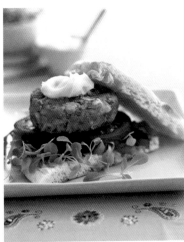 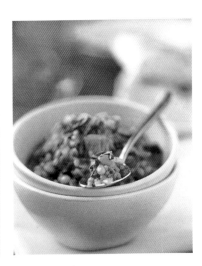

Tagliatelle, peas and herb sauce

375 g (13 oz) dried or 500 g
  (1 lb 2 oz) fresh tagliatelle

250 ml (9 fl oz/1 cup) vegetable stock

2 leeks, white part only, thinly sliced

3 garlic cloves, crushed

235 g (8½ oz/1½ cups) shelled
  fresh peas

1 tbsp finely chopped mint

400 g (14 oz) asparagus spears,
  ends trimmed, cut into 5 cm
  (2 in) lengths

1 large handful flat-leaf (Italian)
  parsley, finely chopped

2 handfuls basil, shredded

80 ml (2½ fl oz/⅓ cup) light cream

pinch of ground nutmeg

1 tbsp grated parmesan cheese

1 tbsp extra virgin olive oil

extra grated parmesan, to garnish
  (optional)

1 Bring a large saucepan of water to the boil and cook the tagliatelle until al dente. Drain well.

2 Put 125 ml (4 fl oz/½ cup) of the stock and the leek in a large, deep frying pan. Cook over low heat, stirring often, for 4–5 minutes. Stir in the garlic, peas and mint and cook for 1 minute. Add the remaining stock and 125 ml (4 fl oz/½ cup) water and bring to the boil, then reduce the heat and simmer for 5 minutes.

3 Add the asparagus, parsley and basil and season well with salt (if desired) and freshly ground black pepper. Simmer for a further 3–4 minutes, or until the asparagus is just tender. Gradually increase the heat to reduce the sauce to a light coating consistency. Stir in the cream, nutmeg and parmesan and adjust the seasoning, to taste.

4 Add the tagliatelle to the sauce and toss lightly to coat. Divide among individual serving bowls and drizzle with the extra virgin olive oil. Garnish with extra grated parmesan, if desired.

Prep time 20 minutes
Cooking time 25 minutes
Serves 4

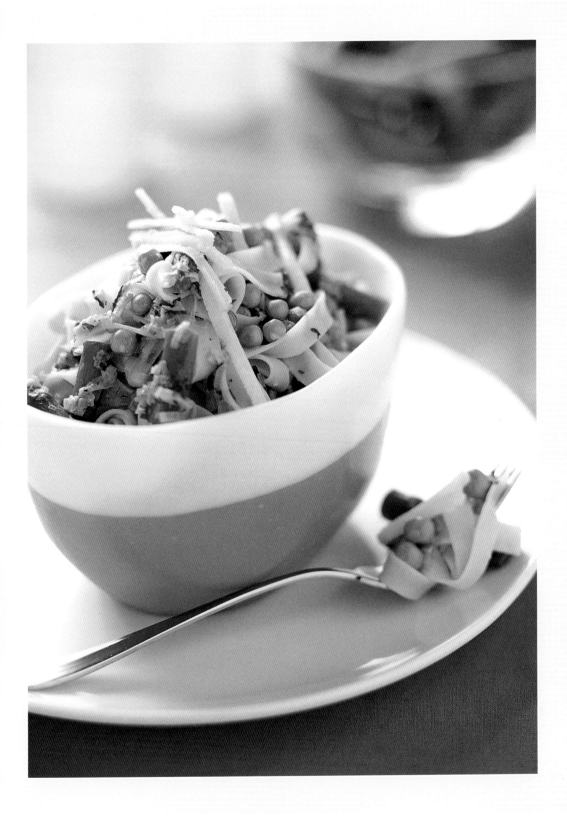

Lentil and vegetable curry

1 tsp canola oil

1 large onion, chopped

2 garlic cloves, chopped

1–2 tbsp curry paste

1 tsp ground turmeric

200 g (7 oz/1 cup) green lentils, rinsed and drained

1.25 litres (44 fl oz/5 cups) vegetable stock or water

1 large carrot, peeled and cut into 2 cm (³⁄₄ in) cubes

2 potatoes, peeled and cut into 2 cm (³⁄₄ in) cubes

250 g (9 oz) sweet potato, peeled and cut into 2 cm (³⁄₄ in) cubes

350 g (12 oz) cauliflower, broken into small florets

150 g (5½ oz) green beans, trimmed and halved

basil, to serve

coriander (cilantro) leaves, to serve

1 Heat the oil in a saucepan over medium heat. Add the onion and garlic and cook for 3 minutes, or until softened. Stir in the curry paste and turmeric and cook for 1 minute. Add the lentils and stock or water and bring to the boil. Reduce the heat, cover and simmer for 30 minutes, then add the carrot, potato and sweet potato. Simmer, covered, for a further 20 minutes, or until the lentils and vegetables are tender.

2 Add the cauliflower and beans, then cover and simmer for 10 minutes, or until the vegetables are cooked and most of the liquid has been absorbed. Remove the lid and simmer for a few minutes if there is still too much liquid remaining.

3 Divide the curry among the serving bowls and top with basil and coriander leaves. Serve with basmati rice.

Prep time 20 minutes
Cooking time 1 hour 10 minutes
Serves 4

nutrition per serve Energy **1986 kJ (474 Cal)** Fat **13.3 g** Saturated fat **1.9 g**
Protein **13.4 g** Carbohydrate **59.4 g** Fibre **16.9 g** Cholesterol **0 mg** Sodium **1175 mg**

Pearl barley and mushroom pilaff

330 g (11½ oz/1½ cups) pearl barley

3 dried shiitake mushrooms

625 ml (21½ fl oz/2½ cups) vegetable stock

125 ml (4 fl oz/½ cup) dry sherry

2 tbsp olive oil

1 large onion, finely chopped

3 garlic cloves, crushed

2 tbsp grated fresh ginger

1 tsp sichuan peppercorns, crushed

500 g (1 lb 2 oz) mixed fresh Asian mushrooms (oyster, Swiss brown, enoki)

500 g (1 lb 2 oz) choy sum (Chinese flowering cabbage), cut into short lengths

3 tsp kecap manis

1 tsp sesame oil

Prep time 20 minutes + overnight soaking

Cooking time 45 minutes

Serves 4

1 Soak the barley in enough cold water to cover for at least 6 hours, or preferably overnight. Drain. Soak the shiitake mushrooms in enough boiling water to cover for 15 minutes. Strain, reserving 125 ml (4 fl oz/½ cup) of the soaking liquid. Discard the stalks and thinly slice the mushroom caps.

2 Heat the stock and sherry in a small saucepan. Cover and keep at a low simmer.

3 Heat the oil in a large saucepan over medium heat and cook the onion for 4–5 minutes, or until softened. Add the garlic, ginger and peppercorns and cook for 1 minute. Slice the fresh Asian mushrooms, reserving the enoki, if using, for later. Increase the heat, add the mushrooms and cook for 5 minutes, or until softened. Add the barley, shiitake, reserved soaking liquid and hot stock and stir to combine. Bring to the boil, then reduce the heat to low and simmer, covered, for 35 minutes, or until the liquid evaporates.

4 Steam the choy sum until just wilted. Add the choy sum to the barley mixture along with the enoki mushrooms. Stir in the kecap manis and sesame oil and serve hot.

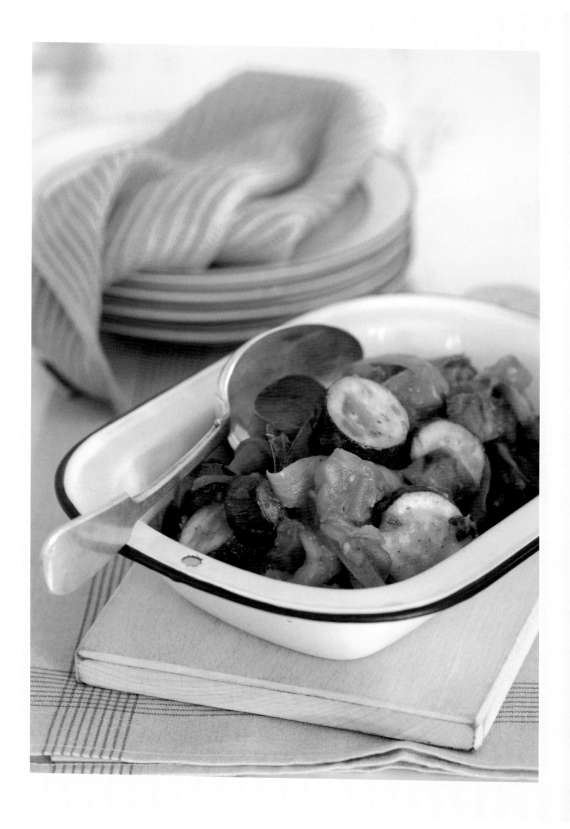

nutrition per serve   Energy **1545 kJ (369 Cal)**   Fat **12.9 g**   Saturated fat **1.7 g**
Protein **11.5 g**   Carbohydrate **46.7 g**   Fibre **9.9 g**   Cholesterol **<1 mg**   Sodium **402 mg**

Ratatouille

250 g (9 oz) eggplant (aubergine)

2 tbsp olive oil

250 g (9 oz) zucchini (courgettes),
    thickly sliced

2 onions, cut into wedges

1 red capsicum (pepper), cut into
    bite-sized cubes

1 green capsicum (pepper), cut into
    bite-sized cubes

2 garlic cloves, crushed

500 g (1 lb 2 oz) ripe tomatoes,
    chopped

1 tbsp chopped parsley

4 wholegrain bread rolls, to serve

Prep time 20 minutes +
15 minutes standing
Cooking time 40 minutes
Serves 4

1   Thickly slice eggplant, then spread it in a colander and sprinkle liberally with salt. Leave for 15 minutes, then rinse, pat dry with paper towels and cut into cubes.

2   Heat 1½ tablespoons of the oil in a large frying pan. Add the eggplant and zucchini in batches and cook for a few minutes, or until lightly browned. Drain well on paper towels.

3   Add the remaining oil to the pan and cook the onion over low heat for 3 minutes, or until golden. Add the red and green capsicums and cook for 5 minutes, or until tender but not browned. Add the garlic and tomatoes and cook, stirring, for 5 minutes.

4   Stir in the eggplant and the zucchini. Leave to simmer for 15–20 minutes to reduce and thicken the sauce. Stir in the parsley, and then season to taste with salt (if desired) and freshly ground black pepper. Serve with the wholegrain bread rolls.

Tempeh stir-fry

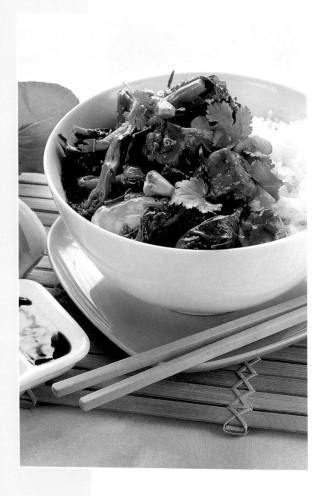

400 g (14 oz/2 cups) basmati rice, rinsed and drained

1 tsp sesame oil

2 tsp peanut oil

2 garlic cloves, crushed

1 tbsp grated fresh ginger

1 red chilli, thinly sliced

4 spring onions (scallions), sliced on the diagonal

300 g (10½ oz) tempeh, diced

500 g (1 lb 2 oz) baby bok choy (pak choy) leaves

nutrition per serve
Energy **2917 kJ (697 Cal)** Fat **17.9 g** Saturated fat **3.3 g** Protein **29.6 g** Carbohydrate **100.3 g** Fibre **14.4 g** Cholesterol **0 mg** Sodium **695 mg**

800 g (1 lb 12 oz/1 bunch) Chinese broccoli (gai larn), chopped

125 ml (4 fl oz/½ cup) mushroom oyster sauce

2 tbsp rice vinegar

2 tbsp chopped coriander (cilantro) leaves

40 g (1½ oz/¼ cup) cashew nuts, toasted

Prep time 15 minutes

Cooking time 30 minutes

Serves 4

1 Put the rice and 1 litre (35 fl oz/4 cups) water in a saucepan and bring to the boil over medium heat. Reduce the heat to low, cover and cook for 20 minutes, or until the rice is tender. Remove from the heat and set aside, covered, for 5 minutes.

2 Meanwhile, heat a wok until very hot, add the sesame and peanut oils and swirl to coat. Reduce the heat to medium, add the garlic, ginger, chilli and spring onion and cook for 1–2 minutes, or until the spring onion is soft. Add the tempeh and cook for 5 minutes, or until golden. Remove from the wok and keep warm.

3 Add half the bok choy, half the Chinese broccoli and 1 tablespoon water to the wok and cook, covered, for 3–4 minutes, or until the greens are wilted. Remove and repeat with the remaining greens and more water.

4 Return the greens and tempeh to the wok, add the mushroom oyster sauce and vinegar and warm through. Top with the coriander and nuts and serve with rice.

nutrition per serve   Energy **1994 kJ (476 Cal)** Fat **6.2 g** Saturated fat **1 g**
Protein **18 g** Carbohydrate **81.7 g** Fibre **11.7 g** Cholesterol **<1 mg** Sodium **934 mg**

Bean burgers and salad

425 g (15 oz) tin cannellini beans or butter beans, drained and rinsed

olive oil spray

1 onion, finely chopped

2 garlic cloves, finely chopped

1 green chilli, seeded and finely chopped

1 tsp ground cumin

1 zucchini (courgette), grated

1 carrot, grated

80 g (2¾ oz/1 cup) fresh wholegrain breadcrumbs

2 tsp olive oil

2 handfuls mixed salad leaves

225 g (8 oz) tin sliced beetroot, drained

2 large ripe tomatoes, sliced

1 loaf Turkish pide bread, cut into 4 slices, then sliced horizontally

4 tbsp low-fat mayonnaise

1 Mash the beans with a fork and place in a large bowl. Spray a heavy-based frying pan with the oil. Add the onion, garlic and chilli and cook for 3 minutes, or until softened. Stir in the cumin and transfer the onion mixture to the bowl with the beans.

2 Add the grated zucchini, carrot and breadcrumbs to the bowl. Use clean hands to mix the ingredients. Form into four balls, then flatten to 10 cm (4 in) patties. Cover and refrigerate for at least 20 minutes.

3 Heat a heavy-based non-stick frying pan over medium heat and add the olive oil. Cook the patties over medium heat for 2–3 minutes on each side, or until golden and heated through. Spray each side of the patties with oil as you cook them.

4 To serve, arrange the salad leaves, beetroot and tomato slices on each bread base. Add a bean patty and some mayonnaise and place the remaining bread half on top.

Prep time 20 minutes +
20 minutes refrigeration
Cooking time 10 minutes
Serves 4

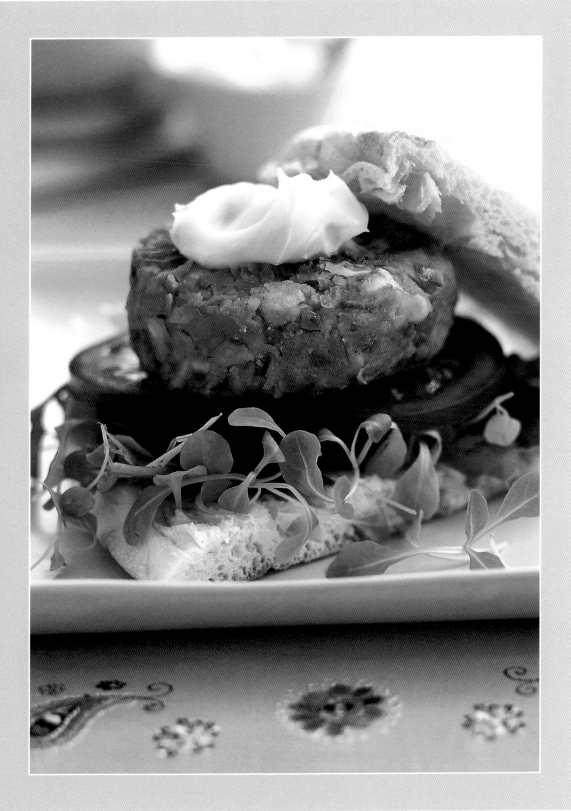

Vegetarian chilli

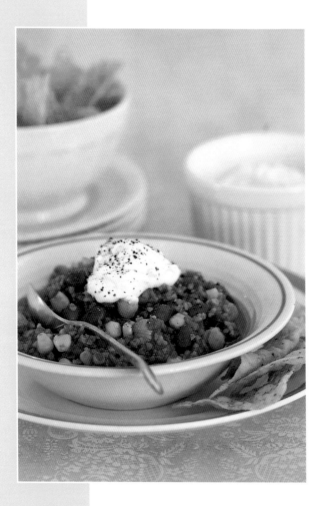

130 g (4½ oz/¾ cup) burghul (bulgur)

250 ml (9 fl oz/1 cup) hot water

2 tsp olive oil

1 large onion, finely chopped

2 garlic cloves, crushed

1 tsp chilli powder

2 tsp ground cumin

1 tsp cayenne pepper

½ tsp ground cinnamon

2 x 400 g (14 oz) tins chopped tomatoes

750 ml (26 fl oz/3 cups) reduced-salt vegetable stock

nutrition per serve
Energy **2086 kJ (498 Cal)** Fat **7.2 g** Saturated fat **1.1 g** Protein **22.7 g** Carbohydrate **72.3 g** Fibre **24.4 g** Cholesterol **0 mg** Sodium **1477 mg**

2 x 400 g (14 oz) tins red kidney beans, drained and rinsed

2 x 300 g (10½ oz) tins chickpeas, drained and rinsed

310 g (11 oz) tin corn kernels, drained

2 tbsp tomato paste (concentrated purée)

3 tbsp chopped parsley

Prep time 10 minutes + 10 minutes soaking

Cooking time 40 minutes

Serves 4

1 Put the burghul in a bowl, cover with the hot water and soak for 10 minutes.

2 Heat the oil in a large saucepan over medium heat and cook the onion for 10 minutes, stirring often, until soft and golden. Add the garlic, chilli powder, cumin, cayenne pepper and cinnamon and cook, stirring, for a further minute.

3 Add the tomatoes, stock and burghul. Bring to the boil, then reduce the heat and simmer for 10 minutes. Stir in the kidney beans, chickpeas, corn and tomato paste and simmer for 20 minutes, stirring often. Garnish with the parsley. If desired, top with a little low-fat plain yoghurt or sour cream, or grated low-fat cheddar cheese. For a special treat, serve with baked corn chips.

Spiced lentil and rice pilaff

200 g (7 oz/1 cup) puy lentils or
   tiny blue-green lentils

2 tsp olive oil

1 small red chilli, seeded and
   chopped

2 garlic cloves, chopped

2 tsp grated fresh ginger

1 red onion, chopped

1 small red capsicum (pepper),
   chopped

1 tsp garam masala

1 tsp ground turmeric

150 g (5½ oz/¾ cup) brown
   basmati rice

1 litre (35 fl oz/4 cups) hot vegetable
   stock or water

155 g (5½ oz/1 cup) frozen peas,
   thawed

1 Put the lentils in a bowl, cover with water and soak for 1 hour. Drain.

2 Heat the oil in a deep heavy-based frying pan. Add the chilli, garlic and ginger and cook for 1 minute, then add the onion and capsicum. Cook, stirring, for 2–3 minutes, or until softened. Add the garam masala and turmeric and cook, stirring, for 1 minute.

3 Stir in the lentils, rice and hot stock or water. Continue stirring and bring to the boil, then reduce the heat, cover and simmer for 40 minutes, or until the lentils and rice are cooked. Stir in the peas and heat through. Serve with a mixed salad.

Prep time 10 minutes +
1 hour soaking

Cooking time 45 minutes

Serves 4

Pumpkin and broad bean risotto

350 g (12 oz) peeled pumpkin (winter squash)

olive oil spray

750 ml (26 fl oz/3 cups) vegetable stock

1 tbsp olive oil

1 large onion, finely chopped

2 garlic cloves, finely chopped

220 g (7¾ oz/1 cup) arborio rice

200 g (7 oz) Swiss brown mushrooms, halved

310 g (11 oz/2 cups) frozen broad (fava) beans,
    thawed, peeled

4 tbsp grated parmesan cheese

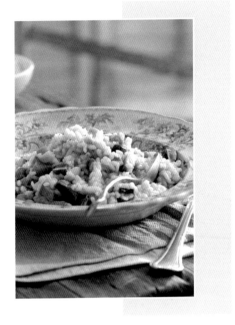

1   Preheat oven to 200°C (400°F/Gas 6). Cut pumpkin into
    small chunks, put in a roasting tin and spray with oil.
    Bake for 20 minutes or until tender. Cover and set aside.

2   Put the stock in a saucepan, bring to the boil, then
    reduce the heat to low and keep at simmering point.

3   Heat oil in a frying pan. Add onion and garlic, cover, and
    cook for 10 minutes over low heat. Add rice and cook,
    stirring, for 2 minutes. Stir in 125 ml (4 fl oz/½ cup) of
    stock and stir rice until stock has been absorbed. Stir in
    125 ml (4 fl oz/½ cup) of stock. When stock is absorbed,
    add mushrooms and remaining stock, a little at a time,
    until it is absorbed and rice is tender.

4   Stir in pumpkin and broad beans to heat through. Divide
    risotto among serving bowls, season with black pepper
    and sprinkle with grated parmesan.

Prep time 35 minutes
Cooking time 1 hour
Serves 4

nutrition per serve   Energy **1661 kJ (397 Cal)** Fat **9.4 g** Saturated fat **1.4 g**
Protein **15.6 g** Carbohydrate **57.6 g** Fibre **12 g** Cholesterol **0 mg** Sodium **875 mg**

Vegetarian paella

200 g (7 oz/1 cup) dried haricot (navy) beans

¼ tsp saffron threads

2 tbsp olive oil

1 onion, diced

1 red capsicum (pepper), thinly sliced

5 garlic cloves, crushed

275 g (9¾ oz/1¼ cups) paella or arborio rice

1 tbsp sweet paprika

½ tsp mixed (pumpkin pie) spice

750 ml (26 fl oz/3 cups) vegetable stock

400 g (14 oz) tin diced tomatoes

1½ tbsp tomato paste (concentrated purée)

150 g (5½ oz/1 cup) tinned or frozen soya beans

100 g (3½ oz) silverbeet (Swiss chard) leaves (no stems), shredded

400 g (14 oz) tin artichoke hearts, drained and quartered

4 tbsp chopped coriander (cilantro) leaves

1 Put the haricot beans in a bowl, cover with cold water and leave to soak overnight. Drain and rinse well.

2 Put the saffron threads in a small frying pan over medium–low heat. Dry-fry, shaking the pan, for 1 minute, or until darkened. Remove from the heat and when cool, crumble into a small bowl. Pour in 125 ml (4 fl oz/½ cup) warm water and set aside to steep.

3 Heat the oil in a large paella pan or frying pan. Add the onion and capsicum and cook over medium–high heat for 5 minutes, or until the onion softens. Stir in the garlic and cook for 1 minute. Reduce the heat and add the drained beans, rice, paprika, mixed spice and ½ teaspoon salt (if desired). Stir to coat. Add the saffron water, stock, tomatoes and tomato paste and bring to the boil. Cover, reduce the heat and simmer for 20 minutes.

4 Stir in the soya beans, silverbeet and artichoke hearts and cook, covered, for 8 minutes, or until all the liquid has been absorbed and the rice and beans are tender. Turn off the heat and leave for 5 minutes. Stir in the coriander just before serving.

Prep time 20 minutes + overnight soaking
Cooking time 40 minutes
Serves 6

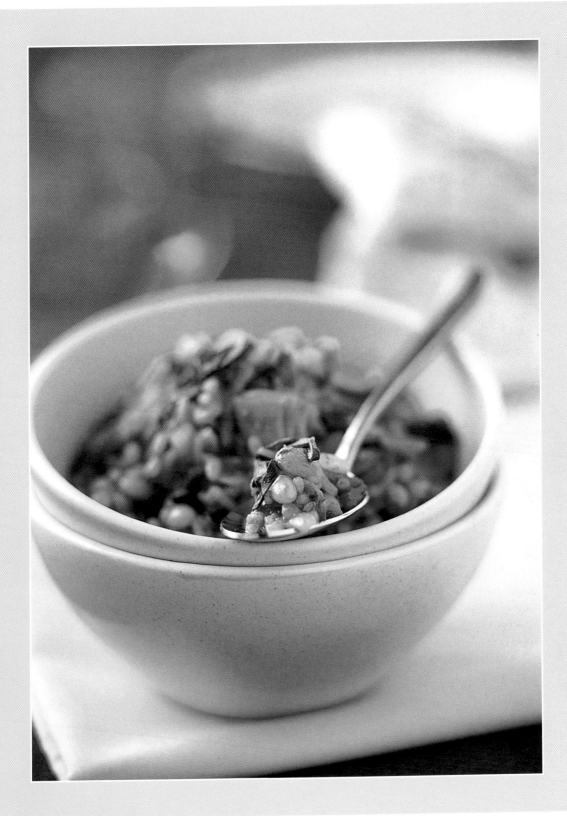

Spinach cannelloni

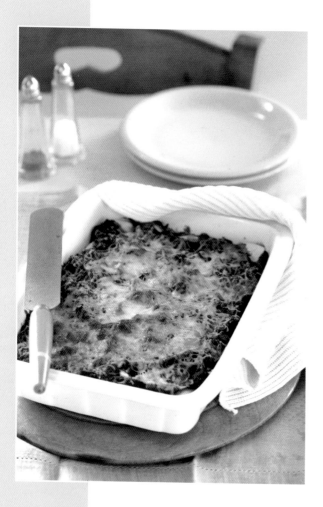

1 tbsp olive oil

2 large onions, chopped

4 garlic cloves, crushed

1 kg (2 lb 4 oz) English spinach, washed, finely chopped

650 g (1 lb 7 oz/2⅔ cups) low-fat ricotta cheese

2 eggs, lightly beaten

pinch of freshly grated nutmeg

olive oil spray

2 x 400 g (14 oz) tins chopped tomatoes

125 ml (4 fl oz/½ cup) dry white wine

2 tbsp tomato paste (concentrated purée)

1 tsp soft brown sugar

2 tbsp chopped basil

250 g (9 oz) dried cannelloni tubes

110 g (3¾ oz/¾ cup) grated reduced-fat mozzarella cheese

35 g (1¼ oz/⅓ cup) grated parmesan cheese

nutrition per serve Energy **2008 kJ (480 Cal)** Fat **16.4 g** Saturated fat **6.3 g**
Protein **31.2 g** Carbohydrate **43.5 g** Fibre **9 g** Cholesterol **82 mg** Sodium **506 mg**

Prep time 45 minutes

Cooking time 1½ hours

Serves 6

1   Heat 2 teaspoons of the oil in a large saucepan. Add half the onion and cook for 3 minutes, then stir in half the garlic and cook for 1 minute. Add the chopped spinach and cook for 2 minutes. Cover the pan and steam the spinach for 1–2 minutes, or until wilted. Set aside to cool slightly. Transfer to a colander and squeeze to remove the moisture.

2   Mix the spinach with the ricotta, eggs and nutmeg. Season with salt (if desired) and freshly ground black pepper. Preheat oven to 180°C (350°F/Gas 4) and spray a large 35 x 24 x 5 cm (14 x 9½ x 2 in) ovenproof dish with oil.

3   To make the sauce, heat the remaining oil in a large frying pan and cook the remaining onion over low heat for 5 minutes, then add the remaining garlic and cook for 1 minute. Add the tomatoes, wine, tomato paste, sugar and basil. Bring to the boil, then reduce the heat and simmer for 30 minutes.

4   Spread one-third of the tomato sauce in the dish. Spoon 2–3 tablespoons of the spinach mixture into each cannelloni tube and arrange neatly in the dish. Spoon the remaining sauce over the top and sprinkle with mozzarella and parmesan. Bake for 40–45 minutes, or until the cannelloni is tender and the top is crisp and golden. Serve with a green salad.

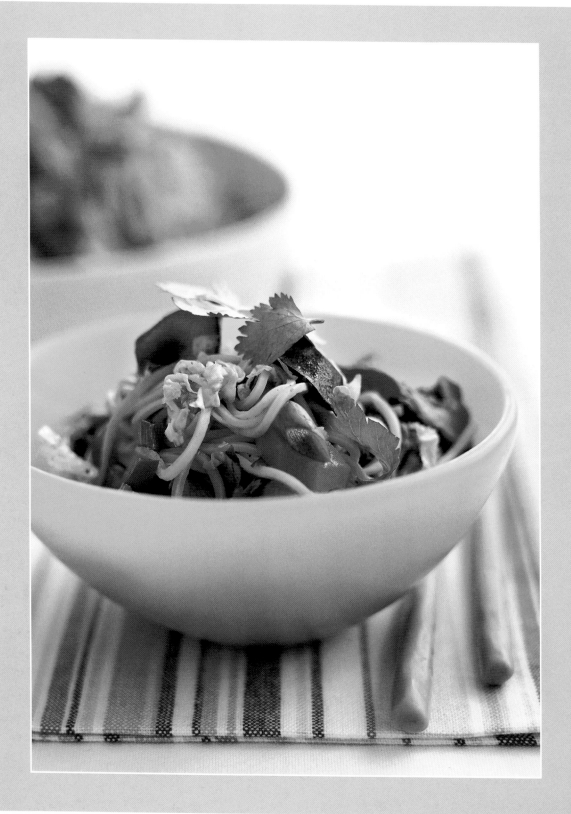

nutrition per serve   Energy **1692 kJ (404 Cal)**   Fat **9.6 g**   Saturated fat **1.2 g**
Protein **23.3 g**   Carbohydrate **46.3 g**   Fibre **11.4 g**   Cholesterol **9 mg**   Sodium **526 mg**

Stir-fry with egg noodles

200 g (7 oz) dried egg noodles

2 tsp canola oil

8 spring onions (scallions), cut
　　into 2.5 cm (1 in) lengths

3 cm (1¼ in) square piece fresh
　　ginger, cut into thin matchsticks

2 garlic cloves, crushed

200 g (7 oz) Swiss brown
　　mushrooms, quartered

1 red capsicum (pepper), thinly
　　sliced

1 zucchini (courgette), cut on the
　　diagonal into 1 cm (½ in) slices

1 carrot, thinly sliced on the
　　diagonal

300 g (10½ oz) broccoli florets

300 g (10½ oz) Chinese cabbage
　　(wong bok), shredded

2 tbsp hoisin sauce

3 tbsp sake or dry sherry

300 g (10½ oz) packet firm tofu,
　　drained and cut into cubes

1 handful coriander (cilantro) leaves,
　　plus extra, to serve

1   Bring a large saucepan of water to the boil. Add the noodles and cook for 5 minutes, or until tender. Drain.

2   Heat a wok over high heat, add the oil and swirl to coat. Add the spring onion and ginger to the wok and stir-fry for 1 minute. Add the garlic and mushrooms and cook for 1 minute, then add the capsicum, zucchini, carrot and broccoli and stir-fry for 3–4 minutes. Pour in 1–2 tablespoons water to help steam the vegetables, if necessary. Add the cabbage, hoisin sauce and sake and stir-fry for 2–3 minutes, or until the cabbage has wilted and all the ingredients are well combined.

3   Toss in the tofu, noodles and coriander and gently stir until well coated in the sauce. Serve immediately sprinkled with extra coriander leaves.

Prep time 20 minutes

Cooking time 15 minutes

Serves 4

nutrition per serve   Energy **1100 kJ (263 Cal)** Fat **10.7 g** Saturated fat **1.4 g**
Protein **10.8 g** Carbohydrate **27.1 g** Fibre **8.8 g** Cholesterol **3 mg** Sodium **76 mg**

Stuffed eggplants

60 g (2¼ oz/⅓ cup) brown lentils

2 large eggplants (aubergines)

olive oil spray

1 red onion, chopped

2 garlic cloves, crushed

1 red capsicum (pepper), finely
    chopped

40 g (1½ oz/¼ cup) pine nuts,
    toasted

440 g (15½ oz) tin chopped tomatoes

140 g (5 oz/¾ cup) cooked
    short-grain brown rice

2 tbsp chopped coriander (cilantro)
    leaves

1 tbsp chopped parsley

2 tbsp grated parmesan cheese

Prep time 20 minutes

Cooking time 1 hour

Serves 4

1 Put lentils in a saucepan, cover with water and simmer for 25 minutes, or until soft. Drain and set aside.

2 Slice the eggplants in half lengthways and scoop out the flesh, leaving a 1 cm (½ in) thick shell. Chop the flesh finely.

3 Spray a deep, large non-stick frying pan with the oil, add 1 tablespoon water to the pan, then add the onion and garlic and stir over medium heat until softened. Add the lentils, capsicum, pine nuts, tomatoes, rice and eggplant flesh and stir over medium heat for 10 minutes, or until the eggplant has softened. Add the coriander and parsley. Season, then toss until well mixed.

4 Cook the eggplant shells in boiling water for 4–5 minutes, or until tender. Spoon the filling into the shells and sprinkle with the parmesan. Place under a preheated grill (broiler) and cook for 5–10 minutes, or until golden. Serve immediately.

nutrition per serve
Energy **1874 kJ (448 Cal)** Fat **10.4 g** Saturated fat **1.4 g** Protein **24.5 g** Carbohydrate **61.8 g** Fibre **9.3 g** Cholesterol **0 mg** Sodium **2150 mg**

Soba noodles with tofu

2 tsp sesame oil

3 tbsp light soy sauce

2 tbsp mirin

2 garlic cloves, finely chopped

2 tsp finely chopped fresh ginger

300 g (10½ oz) packet firm tofu,
   drained and cut into 3 cm (1¼ in)
   cubes

300 g (10½ oz/½ bunch) Chinese
   broccoli (gai larn)

280 g (10 oz) packet soba
   (buckwheat) noodles

115 g (4 oz) fresh baby corn,
   trimmed

1 tsp canola oil

4 red Asian shallots, chopped

150 g (5½ oz) field mushrooms,
   thickly sliced

2 tsp sesame seeds, lightly toasted

1 Combine the sesame oil, soy sauce, mirin, garlic and ginger in a large non-metallic bowl. Add the tofu and gently coat in the marinade. Set aside for at least 15 minutes.

2 Trim the Chinese broccoli, wash and drain, then cut into 5 cm (2 in) pieces. Set aside.

3 Put the soba noodles in a large saucepan of cold water and bring to the boil. Add 250 ml (9 fl oz/1 cup) cold water, bring to the boil again and cook for 5 minutes. Drain. Blanch the corn in a saucepan of boiling water for 2 minutes, refresh in cold water and drain.

4 Heat the oil in a large non-stick wok. Add the shallots and mushrooms and stir-fry for 2–3 minutes. Add the Chinese broccoli and corn to the wok with 80 ml (2½ fl oz/⅓ cup) water. Stir-fry for a further 2 minutes, or until the Chinese broccoli is just wilted. Add the tofu and marinade and gently stir-fry until combined and heated through. Scatter with sesame seeds and serve on a bed of soba noodles.

Prep time 15 minutes +
15 minutes marinating

Cooking time 15 minutes

Serves 4

Vegetable tagine

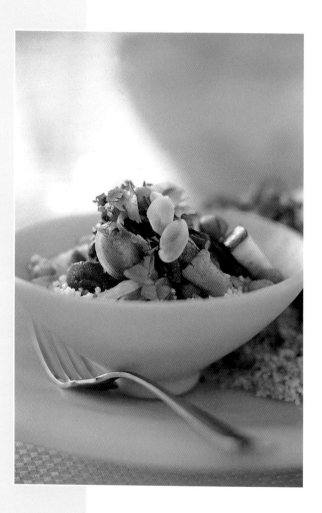

4 ripe tomatoes

¼ tsp saffron threads

2 tbsp flaked almonds

2 tbsp olive oil

2 onions, thinly sliced

3 garlic cloves, crushed

2 thin carrots, cut into 5 mm
(¼ in) slices

1 cinnamon stick

2 tsp ground cumin

1 tsp ground ginger

½ tsp ground turmeric

½ tsp cayenne pepper

300 g (10½ oz) peeled pumpkin
(winter squash), cut into 2 cm
(¾ in) cubes

400 g (14 oz) tin chickpeas,
drained and rinsed

nutrition per serve
Energy **2149 kJ (513 Cal)** Fat **11.3 g** Saturated fat **1.7 g**
Protein **16.8 g** Carbohydrate **82.3 g** Fibre **7.1 g** Cholesterol **0 mg** Sodium **1172 mg**

500 ml (17 fl oz/2 cups) vegetable
  stock

1 zucchini (courgette), halved
  lengthways, then cut into 1 cm
  (½ in) slices

4 tbsp raisins

50 g (1¾ oz/½ bunch) coriander
  (cilantro) leaves, roughly chopped

Couscous

625 ml (21½ fl oz/2½ cups)
  vegetable stock

465 g (1 lb/2½ cups) couscous

2 tsp reduced-fat margarine

Prep time 25 minutes
Cooking time 50 minutes
Serves 6

1 To peel the tomatoes, score a cross in the base of each
tomato. Put in a heatproof bowl and cover with boiling
water. Leave for 30 seconds, then transfer to cold water
and peel the skin away from the cross. To seed, cut the
tomatoes in half and scoop out the seeds with a
teaspoon. Cut the tomatoes into quarters.

2 Dry-fry the saffron threads in a small frying pan over
low heat for 1 minute, until darkened. Remove from the
heat and cool. Repeat with the almonds, then remove
and set aside.

3 Heat the oil in a large flameproof casserole dish.
Add the onion, garlic, carrot, cinnamon stick, cumin,
ginger, turmeric, cayenne pepper and saffron. Cook over
medium–low heat, stirring often, for 10 minutes. Add
the tomatoes, pumpkin and chickpeas and stir to coat.
Add the stock and bring to the boil. Cover and simmer
for 10 minutes. Stir in the zucchini, raisins and half the
coriander. Cover and simmer for a further 20 minutes.

4 To make the couscous, bring the stock to the boil in a
large saucepan. Put the couscous in a large heatproof
bowl and pour over the hot stock. Cover and leave for
5 minutes, then fluff the grains with a fork. Stir in the
margarine and season.

5 Spoon the couscous into serving bowls. Discard the
cinnamon sticks and then spoon the vegetables and
sauce over the couscous and sprinkle with the toasted
almonds and the remaining coriander. Serve at once.

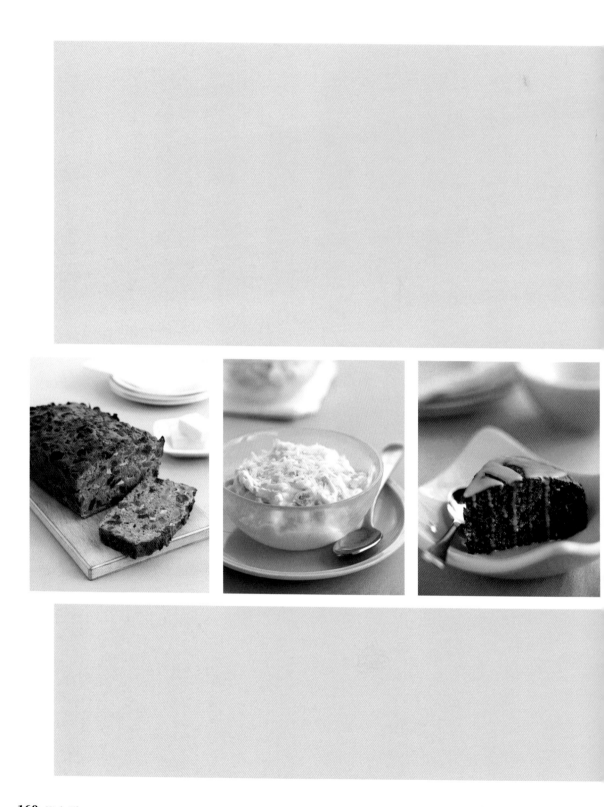

Sweet things

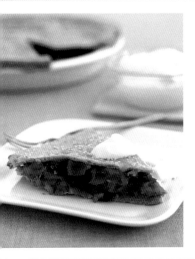 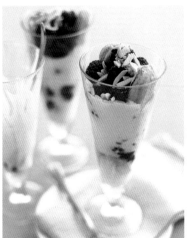 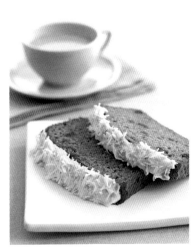

nutrition per serve   Energy **1165 kJ (278 Cal)** Fat **7 g** Saturated fat **0.8 g**
Protein **13 g** Carbohydrate **34.7 g** Fibre **8.6 g** Cholesterol **38 mg** Sodium **132 mg**

Yoghurt and savoiardi parfait

750 g (1 lb 10 oz/3 cups) low-fat
   plain yoghurt

55 g (2 oz/¼ cup) sugar

10 passionfruit

125 g (4½ oz) savoiardi (sponge
   finger biscuits), cut to fit
   parfait glasses

375 g (13 oz/3 cups) fresh or frozen
   raspberries

60 g (2¼ oz/½ cup) slivered
   almonds, toasted

1 Put the yoghurt, sugar and passionfruit pulp in a bowl
and mix well to combine. Divide one-third of the
mixture among six 250 ml (9 fl oz/1 cup) parfait glasses.

2 Top the yoghurt mixture with a layer of savoiardi
biscuits, then with a layer of raspberries.

3 Repeat with another layer of yoghurt, biscuits and
raspberries, and top with a layer of yoghurt. Top with
the remaining raspberries and the toasted almonds.
Refrigerate for 1 hour before serving.

Prep time 20 minutes +

1 hour refrigeration

Cooking time Nil

Serves 6

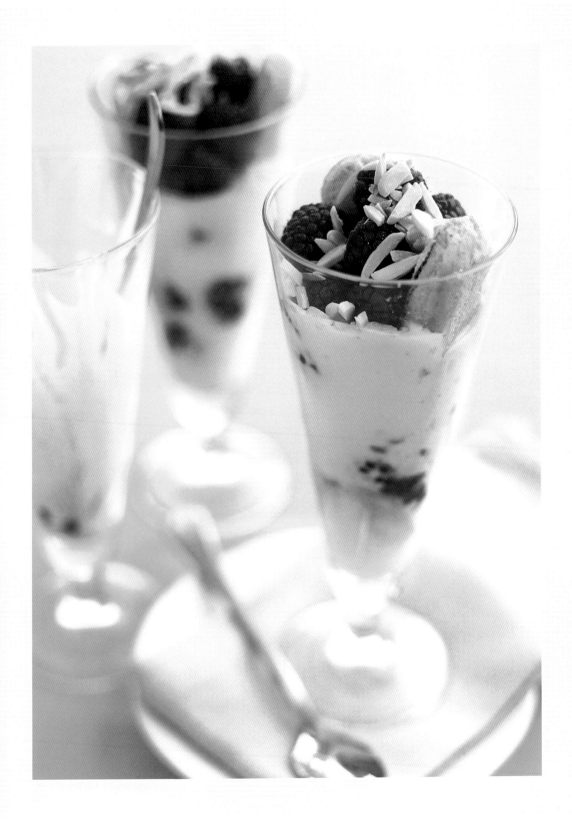

nutrition per serve   Energy **1034 kJ (247 Cal)** Fat **0.6 g** Saturated fat **0.2 g**
Protein **6.3 g** Carbohydrate **53.3 g** Fibre **5.1 g** Cholesterol **4 mg** Sodium **81 mg**

Stewed fruit with custard

2 tbsp blackcurrant syrup

2 large pears, peeled, cored and
    quartered

1 large apple, peeled, cored and
    quartered

500 g (1 lb 2 oz) rhubarb, trimmed,
    cut into 3 cm (1¼ in) pieces

500 ml (17 fl oz/2 cups) skim milk

60 g (2¼ oz/¼ cup) caster
    (superfine) sugar

1½ tbsp custard powder

Prep time 20 minutes

Cooking time 20 minutes

Serves 4

1 Put the syrup, pears, apple and 3 tablespoons water in a
large saucepan and stir to coat the fruit. Cook, covered,
over low heat for 4 minutes (keep the heat low or the
fruit will scorch on the base of the pan). Add the
rhubarb, toss well to combine, then cover and cook for
a further 6–7 minutes, or until the fruit is just tender.
Remove from the heat, cover and set aside.

2 Put the milk and sugar in a saucepan. Bring to the boil,
then reduce the heat and simmer for 3 minutes. Mix the
custard powder with 1 tablespoon water and mix to a
smooth paste. Return the milk to the boil, stir in the
custard powder mixture and whisk constantly until the
mixture boils and thickens and coats the back of a
wooden spoon.

3 Place fruit in serving dishes and drizzle with any liquid
from the bottom of the pan. Serve with warm custard.

nutrition per slice   Energy **922 kJ (220 Cal)** Fat **10.4 g** Saturated fat **2.5 g**
Protein **5 g** Carbohydrate **26.1 g** Fibre **3.8 g** Cholesterol **<1 mg** Sodium **39 mg**

Chocolate fruit and nut slice

canola oil spray

160 g (5½ oz/1 cup) stoneground wholemeal (whole-wheat) self-raising flour

2 tbsp unsweetened cocoa powder

50 g (1¾ oz/½ cup) wholegrain rolled barley

2 tbsp unprocessed oat bran

35 g (1¼ oz/⅓ cup) ground almonds

30 g (1 oz/⅓ cup) desiccated coconut

60 g (2¼ oz/⅓ cup) soft brown sugar

95 g (3½ oz/½ cup) fruit medley, chopped

60 g (2¼ oz/½ cup) walnuts, chopped

90 g (3¼ oz) reduced-fat margarine, just melted

1 tbsp pure maple syrup

250 ml (9 fl oz/1 cup) low-fat milk

icing (confectioners') sugar, to dust

1 Preheat the oven to 180°C (350°F/Gas 4). Spray a 27 x 17 cm (10¾ x 6½ in) shallow baking tin with oil, then line the base with baking paper, leaving the paper overhanging the two long sides.

2 Sift the flour and cocoa into a large bowl, then return any husks to the bowl. Stir in the rolled barley, oat bran, ground almonds, coconut, brown sugar, fruit medley and walnuts. Make a well in the centre.

3 Combine the melted margarine, maple syrup and milk in a small bowl. Add to the flour mixture and stir until well combined. Spread evenly into the prepared tin.

4 Bake for 25 minutes, or until cooked and firm. Leave in the tin to cool, then turn out onto a wire rack to cool completely. Dust with icing sugar and cut into slices. Serve with fresh berries and low-fat yoghurt or fromage frais, if desired.

Prep time 15 minutes
Cooking time 25 minutes
Makes 12 slices

Crêpes with fruit compote

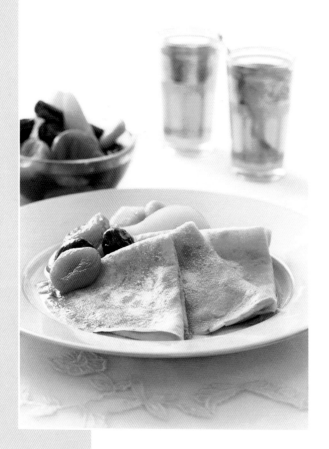

Crêpes

60 g (2¼ oz/½ cup) plain
   (all-purpose) flour

2 eggs

250 ml (9 fl oz/1 cup) skim milk

canola oil spray

2 tsp caster (superfine) sugar

nutrition per serve
Energy **1350 kJ (323 Cal)** Fat **4.1 g** Saturated fat **0.9 g**
Protein **9.2 g** Carbohydrate **56.4 g** Fibre **6.3 g** Cholesterol **96 mg** Sodium **80 mg**

Compote

100 g (3½ oz) whole dried apricots

3 tbsp port or Muscat, or use orange juice

1 vanilla bean, halved lengthways

2 firm pears, peeled, cored and quartered

2 cinnamon sticks

425 g (15 oz) tin pitted prunes in syrup, drained, syrup reserved

Prep time 20 minutes +
30 minutes resting
Cooking time 20 minutes
Serves 4

1 Put the flour in a bowl and gradually add the combined eggs and milk, whisking to remove any lumps. Cover the batter with plastic wrap and set aside for 30 minutes.

2 Meanwhile, to make the compote, put the apricots and port in a saucepan and cook, covered, over low heat for 2–3 minutes, or until softened. Scrape the seeds from the vanilla bean and add the bean and seeds to the pan along with the pear, cinnamon sticks and prune syrup. Simmer, covered, stirring occasionally, for 4 minutes, or until the pear has softened. Add the prunes and simmer for 1 minute.

3 Heat a 20 cm (8 in) non-stick crêpe pan or frying pan over medium heat. Lightly spray with oil. Pour 3 tablespoons of the batter into the pan and swirl evenly over the base. Cook each crêpe for 1 minute, or until the underside is golden. Turn it over and cook the other side for 30 seconds, then remove. Keep warm and repeat to make eight crêpes in total.

4 Fold the crêpes into triangles and sprinkle with the sugar. Serve with the compote.

Energy **1599 kJ (382 Cal)** Fat **8.2 g** Saturated fat **1.6 g**
Protein **7.8 g** Carbohydrate **67.8 g** Fibre **6.2 g** Cholesterol **48 mg** Sodium **81 mg**

Sticky date pudding

280 g (10 oz/1⅔ cups) chopped dates

1 tsp natural vanilla extract

2 tsp bicarbonate of soda (baking soda)

90 g (3¼ oz) reduced-fat margarine

95 g (3½ oz/½ cup) soft brown sugar

2 eggs

150 g (5½ oz/1 cup) wholemeal (whole-wheat) self-raising flour

60 g (2¼ oz/½ cup) self-raising flour

2 tbsp unprocessed oat bran

Sauce

185 ml (6 fl oz/¾ cup) evaporated skim milk

95 g (3½ oz/½ cup) soft brown sugar

1 tbsp margarine

1 tsp custard powder

Prep time 15 minutes
Cooking time 1 hour
Serves 8

1 Preheat the oven to 180°C (350°F/Gas 4). Lightly grease and line base and side of a 20 cm (8 in) round cake tin.

2 Put the dates and 375 ml (13 fl oz/1½ cups) water in a saucepan. Bring to the boil, then reduce the heat and simmer for 5 minutes, or until soft. Stir in the vanilla and bicarbonate of soda and set aside to cool to room temperature.

3 Beat the margarine and sugar with electric beaters until pale and creamy. Gradually add the eggs, beating well after each addition—the mixture may look curdled at this stage, but a spoonful of flour will bring it back together. Fold in the sifted flours (return the husks to the bowl), oat bran and the date mixture in two batches, using a metal spoon.

4 Pour the mixture into the prepared tin. Bake for 50 minutes, or until a skewer comes out clean when inserted into the centre of the pudding. Cool in the tin for 10–15 minutes.

5 To make the sauce, heat the evaporated milk, sugar and margarine in a saucepan until almost boiling. Combine the custard powder and 1 teaspoon water until smooth, then gradually add to the sauce, stirring continually over medium heat until it thickens slightly. Serve warm with the pudding.

Pear and hazelnut bran muffins

250 g (9 oz) dried pears, chopped

120 g (4¼ oz/2 cups) processed
   bran cereal

500 ml (17 fl oz/2 cups) reduced-fat
   milk

310 g (11 oz/1⅓ cups firmly packed)
   soft brown sugar

2 tbsp maple syrup

250 g (9 oz/2 cups) self-raising flour

180 g (6 oz/1¼ cups) hazelnuts,
   roasted and chopped

1 tsp ground cinnamon

1 tsp caster (superfine) sugar

Prep time 10 minutes +
overnight refrigeration
Cooking time 25 minutes
Makes 16

1 Mix the pears, bran cereal, milk, sugar and maple syrup together in a large bowl, then cover and refrigerate overnight.

2 Preheat the oven to 180°C (350°F/Gas 4). Grease 16 regular muffin holes.

3 Sift the flour into the pear and bran cereal mixture and add the nuts. Fold gently until just combined—the batter will be lumpy.

4 Divide the mixture among the muffin holes. Bake for 20–25 minutes, or until the muffins come away from the side of the tin. Cool for 5 minutes, then transfer to a wire rack. Sprinkle with the combined cinnamon and sugar. Serve warm.

nutrition per slice
Energy 1175 kJ (281 Cal) Fat 7.7 g Saturated fat 1 g
Protein 8 g Carbohydrate 43 g Fibre 4.3 g Cholesterol 25 mg Sodium 9 mg

Wholemeal banana bread

olive oil spray

95 g (3½ oz/½ cup) soft brown sugar

1 egg

250 g (9 oz/1 cup) low-fat vanilla fromage frais

2 tbsp canola oil

235 g (8½ oz/1 cup) mashed banana (2 bananas)

30 g (1 oz/¼ cup) pepitas (pumpkin seeds)

60 g (2¼ oz/½ cup) sultanas (golden raisins)

80 g (2¾ oz/½ cup) stoneground self-raising flour

110 g (3¾ oz/⅔ cup) stoneground wholemeal
    (whole-wheat) self-raising flour

½ tsp bicarbonate of soda (baking soda)

3 tbsp unprocessed wheat bran

1 tsp ground cinnamon

½ tsp ground nutmeg

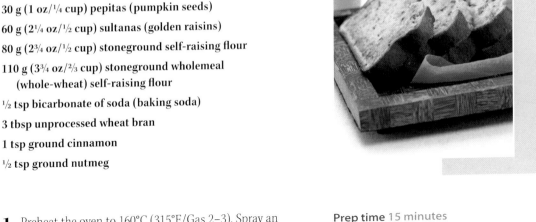

1   Preheat the oven to 160°C (315°F/Gas 2–3). Spray an
    18 x 10 cm (7 x 4 in) loaf (bar) tin with oil and line base
    with baking paper.

2   Put sugar, egg, fromage frais and oil in a bowl and whisk
    until combined. Stir in banana, pepitas and sultanas,
    then fold in sifted flours (return husks to bowl),
    bicarbonate of soda, bran, cinnamon and nutmeg.

3   Spoon mixture into the prepared tin and bake for
    50 minutes, or until cooked through when tested with a
    skewer. Serve warm or cold with low-fat yoghurt or
    fromage frais.

Prep time 15 minutes
Cooking time 50 minutes
Makes 8 slices

Apple pie

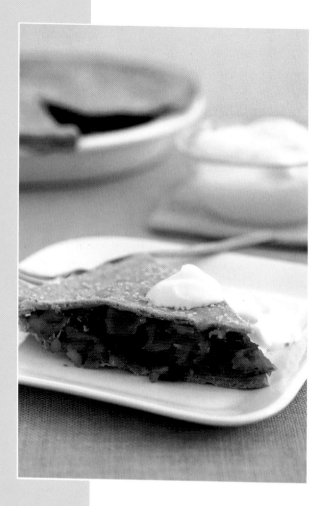

Pastry

canola oil spray

150 g (5½ oz/1 cup) wholemeal
(whole-wheat) flour

125 g (4½ oz/1 cup) plain
(all-purpose) flour

30 g (1 oz/¼ cup) self-raising flour

2 tbsp soft brown sugar

½ tsp ground cinnamon

125 g (4½ oz) reduced-fat margarine,
chilled and chopped

1 egg yolk

3–4 tbsp chilled water

Filling

750 g (1 lb 10 oz) granny smith apples, peeled, cored and sliced (4 large apples)

2 tbsp soft brown sugar

1 tbsp lemon juice

55 g (2 oz/$\frac{1}{3}$ cup) chopped pitted dates

40 g (1$\frac{1}{2}$ oz/$\frac{1}{3}$ cup) raisins

30 g (1 oz/$\frac{1}{4}$ cup) chopped walnuts

milk, to brush

demerara (raw) sugar, to sprinkle

Prep time 40 minutes +
45 minutes refrigeration

Cooking time 1 hour 5 minutes

Serves 8

1 Preheat the oven to 180°C (350°F/Gas 4). Lightly spray an 18 cm (7 in) pie dish with oil.

2 To make the pastry, sift flours into a food processor bowl and return husks to the bowl. Add sugar and cinnamon and briefly pulse. Add margarine and process for 30 seconds. Add egg yolk and 2 tablespoons chilled water and process until the mixture comes together. Add remaining water if necessary to form a soft dough. Gather dough together and lift onto a lightly floured work surface. Press into a ball and flatten slightly. Wrap in plastic and refrigerate for 30 minutes.

3 To make the filling, place apple slices, brown sugar, lemon juice and 2 tablespoons water in a large saucepan, cover and bring to the boil, then reduce heat and simmer for 15 minutes. Stir in dried fruit and walnuts, then leave to cool.

4 Roll out two-thirds of the pastry between two sheets of baking paper. Invert pastry into the dish, allowing any excess to hang over the side, then trim. Cover and refrigerate for 15 minutes. Line pastry shell with a piece of baking paper, pour in baking beads and bake for 10 minutes. Remove paper and baking beads and bake for 10 minutes more. Spoon apple mixture into shell.

5 Roll remaining pastry out to fit the top. Brush the edge of the pastry in dish with water and place pastry lid on top. Trim, then press the edges together. Make several slits in the top of the pie, brush with milk and sprinkle over the sugar. Bake for 30 minutes, or until pastry is crisp and golden. Serve with whipped light cream.

nutrition per muffin

Energy **1065 kJ (254 Cal)** Fat **7 g** Saturated fat **3.7 g** Protein **6.5 g** Carbohydrate **39.3 g** Fibre **6 g** Cholesterol **47 mg** Sodium **26 mg**

Fig and oat bran muffins

125 g (4½ oz/1 cup) self-raising flour

75 g (2½ oz/½ cup) wholemeal (whole-wheat) self-raising flour

½ tsp baking powder

150 g (5½ oz/1 cup) unprocessed oat bran

55 g (2 oz/¼ cup firmly packed) soft brown sugar

250 ml (9 fl oz/1 cup) milk

2 eggs

90 g (3¼ oz/¼ cup) golden syrup or honey

60 g (2¼ oz) unsalted butter, melted and cooled

185 g (6½ oz/1 cup) chopped soft dried figs

3 dried figs, cut into strips, extra

1 Preheat the oven to 200°C (400°F/Gas 6). Grease 12 regular muffin holes.

2 Sift the flours and baking powder into a bowl, return the husks to the bowl, then add the oat bran and sugar. Make a well in the centre.

3 Combine the milk and eggs in a bowl, whisk together and pour into the well. Add the combined golden syrup and melted butter and fold gently until just combined—the batter should be lumpy. Fold in the chopped figs.

4 Divide the mixture among the muffin holes and top with the extra strips of fig. Bake for 20–25 minutes, or until the muffins come away from the side of the tin. Cool in the tin for 5 minutes, then transfer to a wire rack.

Prep time 15 minutes

Cooking time 25 minutes

Makes 12

nutrition per biscuit Energy **503 kJ (120 Cal)** Fat **5.1 g** Saturated fat **1.9 g**
Protein **2.6 g** Carbohydrate **14.9 g** Fibre **2.3 g** Cholesterol **14 mg** Sodium **4 mg**

Oat crunch biscuits

90 g (3¼ oz) unsalted butter,
   softened

95 g (3½ oz/½ cup) soft brown sugar

1 tsp natural vanilla extract

1 egg

140 g (5 oz) apple purée

200 g (7 oz/2 cups) wholegrain
   rolled oats

160 g (5½ oz/1 cup) stoneground
   wholemeal (whole-wheat) self-
   raising flour

75 g (2½ oz/1 cup) lightly crushed
   bran flakes

185 g (6½ oz/1 cup) chopped dried
   apricots

60 g (2¼ oz/½ cup) chopped
   hazelnuts

30 g (1 oz/¼ cup) pepitas
   (pumpkin seeds)

1 Preheat the oven to 190°C (375°F/Gas 5). Lightly grease two large baking trays.

2 Using electric beaters, beat the butter and sugar together until creamy, then add the vanilla and egg and beat well. Stir in the apple purée.

3 Combine the rolled oats, flour, bran flakes, apricots, hazelnuts and pepitas in a large bowl. Stir in the butter mixture until well combined.

4 Place heaped tablespoons of the mixture on the prepared trays and flatten with a spatula to a rough 7 cm (2¾ in) round. Bake for 12–15 minutes, or until the biscuits are cooked through. Cool on a wire cooling rack, then store in an airtight container.

Prep time 20 minutes
Cooking time 15 minutes
Makes 30

nutrition per serve   Energy **884 kJ (211 Cal)** Fat **1.1 g** Saturated fat **0.1 g**
Protein **4.3 g** Carbohydrate **44.1 g** Fibre **6.8 g** Cholesterol **0 mg** Sodium **225 mg**

Summer pudding

150 g (5½ oz) blackcurrants or
   blueberries

150 g (5½ oz) redcurrants

150 g (5½ oz) raspberries

150 g (5½ oz) blackberries

200 g (7 oz) strawberries, hulled and
   quartered or halved

125 g (4½ oz/heaped ½ cup) caster
   (superfine) sugar, or to taste

6–8 slices good-quality sliced white
   bread, crusts removed

Prep time 30 minutes +
overnight refrigeration
Cooking time 5 minutes
Serves 6

1 Put all the berries, except the strawberries, in a large saucepan with 125 ml (4 fl oz/½ cup) water and heat gently for 5 minutes, or until the berries begin to soften. Add the strawberries and remove from the heat. Add the sugar, to taste (how much you need will depend on how ripe the fruit is). Set aside to cool.

2 Line six 170 ml (5½ fl oz/⅔ cup) ovenproof moulds or a 1 litre (35 fl oz/4 cup) pudding basin with the bread. For the small moulds, use one slice of bread for each, cutting a circle of bread to fit the bottom, and strips to fit snugly around the sides. For the basin, cut a large circle out of one slice for the bottom and cut the rest of the bread into wide fingers to fit the side.

3 Drain a little of the juice off the fruit into a bowl. Dip one side of each piece of bread in the juice before fitting it, juice side down, into the mould, leaving no gaps. Do not squeeze or flatten the bread or it won't absorb the juice.

4 Fill the centre of each mould with the fruit and pour in a little juice. Cover the tops with the remaining dipped bread, juice side up, and trim to fit. Cover with plastic wrap. For the small moulds sit a small tin, or a similar weight, on top of each. For the basin, place a small plate that fits inside the basin onto the plastic wrap, then weigh it down with a large tin. Place on an oven tray to catch any juices that may overflow and refrigerate overnight. Carefully turn out the pudding and serve with any leftover fruit mixture. Serve with low-fat cream or ice cream, if desired.

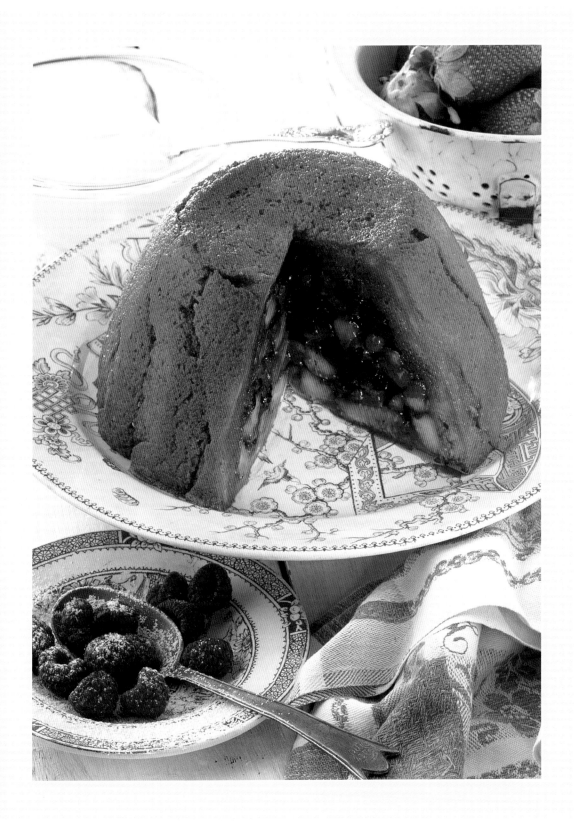

Prune and choc chip biscuits

160 g (5½ oz/1 cup) stoneground
  wholemeal (whole-wheat)
  self-raising flour

50 g (1¾ oz/½ cup) wholegrain
  rolled barley or oats

60 g (2¼ oz/⅓ cup) soft brown sugar

30 g (1 oz/⅓ cup) desiccated coconut

2 tbsp unprocessed oat bran

60 g (2¼ oz/heaped ⅓ cup) dark
  chocolate chips

125 g (4½ oz/½ cup) chopped
  pitted prunes

90 g (3¼ oz) reduced-fat margarine

1 tbsp pure maple syrup

125 ml (4 fl oz/½ cup) buttermilk

2 tsp grated orange zest

1 Preheat the oven to 180°C (350°F/Gas 4). Line a baking tray with baking paper.

2 Sift the flour into a large bowl and return the husks to the bowl. Add the rolled barley, sugar, coconut, oat bran, chocolate chips and prunes. Mix well, separating the prunes with your fingers.

3 Melt the margarine and maple syrup in a small saucepan over low heat. Add the buttermilk and stir in the orange zest. Pour over the flour mixture and combine until moistened.

4 Using 1 heaped tablespoon of batter at a time, drop spoonfuls onto the prepared tray, spacing them evenly apart. Bake for 15 minutes, or until golden brown. Leave on the tray for 2–3 minutes, then transfer to a wire rack to cool completely. The biscuits will crisp on cooling.

Prep time 15 minutes
Cooking time 20 minutes
Makes 16

Fruity bran loaf

olive oil spray

60 g (2¼ oz/1 cup) processed bran cereal

435 ml (15¼ fl oz/1¾ cups) skim milk

380 g (13½ oz/2 cups) dried fruit medley

95 g (3½ oz/½ cup) soft brown sugar

**240 g (8½ oz/1½ cups) stoneground wholemeal
(whole-wheat) self-raising flour**

1 tsp ground cinnamon

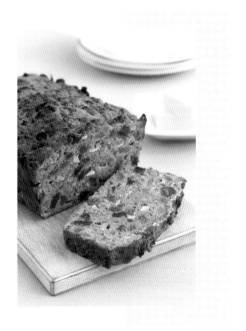

1 Preheat the oven to 180°C (350°F/Gas 4). Spray a
20 x 10 cm (8 x 4 in) loaf (bar) tin with oil and line
the base with baking paper.

2 Put the bran cereal in a large bowl. Stir in the milk, fruit
medley and sugar. Set aside for at least 1 hour to soften
the bran.

3 Meanwhile, sift the flour and cinnamon into a bowl
(return the husks to the bowl). Stir the bran mixture
into the flour and cinnamon. Spoon into the prepared
tin and smooth the surface. Bake for 45–50 minutes, or
until cooked when a skewer inserted into the centre of
the loaf comes out clean. Cool in the tin for 15 minutes,
then turn out. Cut into thick slices to serve.

Prep time 15 minutes +
1 hour soaking
Cooking time 50 minutes
Makes 10 slices

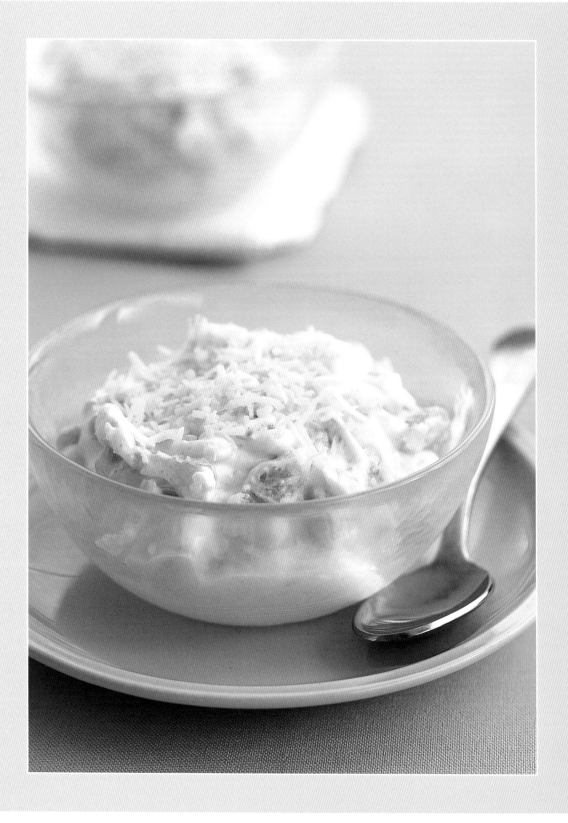

nutrition per serve   Energy **822 kJ (196 Cal)** Fat **2.1 g** Saturated fat **1.7 g**
Protein **4.4 g** Carbohydrate **37.8 g** Fibre **5.9 g** Cholesterol **0 mg** Sodium **64 mg**

Dried apricot fool

30 g (1 oz) finely chopped glacé ginger

210 g (7½ oz) dried apricots, chopped

1 tbsp unprocessed wheat bran

2 egg whites

2 tbsp caster (superfine) sugar

2 tbsp shredded coconut, toasted

Prep time 15 minutes
Cooking time 5 minutes
Serves 4

1 Place the ginger, apricots, wheat bran and 80 ml (2½ fl oz/⅓ cup) water in a small saucepan. Cook, covered, over very low heat for 5 minutes, stirring occasionally. Remove from the heat and allow to cool completely.

2 Using electric beaters, beat the egg whites in a clean dry bowl until soft peaks form. Add the sugar and beat for 3 minutes, or until thick and glossy. Quickly and gently fold the cooled apricot mixture into the egg whites, and divide among four chilled serving glasses. Scatter the coconut over the top and serve immediately.

nutrition per serve
Energy **1380 kJ (330 Cal)** Fat **0.4 g** Saturated fat **<0.1 g** Protein **5.5 g** Carbohydrate **74.1 g** Fibre **7.4 g** Cholesterol **2 mg** Sodium **97 mg**

Fruit in orange ginger syrup

60 g (2¼ oz/¼ cup) caster (superfine) sugar

3 tbsp orange juice

2 strips orange peel

1 cinnamon stick

250 g (9 oz) dried fruit salad, large pieces cut in half

100 g (3½ oz) stoned dates

1 tsp grated fresh ginger

200 g (7 oz) low-fat plain yoghurt

Prep time 10 minutes

Cooking time 10 minutes

Serves 4

1　Put the sugar, orange juice, orange peel, cinnamon stick and 375 ml (13 fl oz/1½ cups) water in a large saucepan. Stir over low heat until the sugar dissolves, then increase the heat and simmer, without stirring, for 5 minutes, or until the syrup has thickened slightly.

2　Add the dried fruit salad, dates and ginger and toss well. Cover and simmer over low heat for 5 minutes, or until the fruit has softened. Remove the pan from the heat and set aside, covered, for 5 minutes. Discard the orange peel and cinnamon stick. If serving cold, remove the fruit from the saucepan and set aside to cool.

3　Place the fruit in individual serving dishes, top with the yoghurt and drizzle a little of the syrup over the top. Serve immediately.

nutrition per serve Energy **1054 kJ (252 Cal)** Fat **4.5 g** Saturated fat **2.8 g**
Protein **1.2 g** Carbohydrate **51 g** Fibre **5.8 g** Cholesterol **13 mg** Sodium **5 mg**

Baked fig and raisin apples

4 large cooking apples

80 g (2¾ oz/⅓ cup firmly packed) soft brown sugar

1½ tbsp chopped raisins

2 dried figs, chopped

½ tsp ground cinnamon (optional)

20 g (¾ oz) unsalted butter

low-fat yoghurt or ricotta cream, to serve

1 Preheat the oven to 220°C (425°F/Gas 7). Core the apples and score the skin around the middle, so the apples won't burst while they are baking.

2 Combine the sugar, raisins, figs and cinnamon, if using. Place each apple on a piece of heavy-duty foil and fill the cavity with the fruit filling. Spread a little butter over the top of each apple, then wrap the foil securely around the apples. Bake for about 40 minutes, or until cooked through. Serve with yoghurt or ricotta cream.

Prep time 10 minutes

Cooking time 40 minutes

Serves 4

Carrot cake

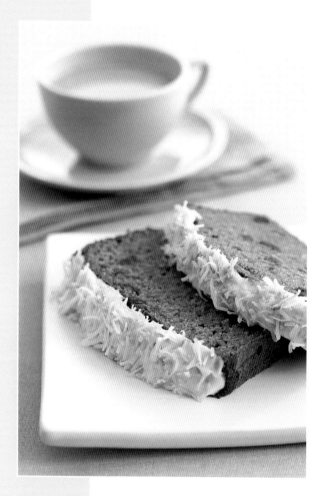

160 g (5½ oz/1 cup) stoneground wholemeal (whole-wheat) self-raising flour

160 g (5½ oz/1 cup) stoneground self-raising flour

1 tsp bicarbonate of soda (baking soda)

2 tsp ground cinnamon

1 tsp mixed (pumpkin pie) spice

75 g (2½ oz/½ cup) unprocessed oat bran

95 g (3½ oz/½ cup) soft brown sugar

60 g (2¼ oz/½ cup) sultanas (golden raisins)

2 eggs, lightly beaten

2 tbsp canola oil

80 ml (2½ fl oz/⅓ cup) skim or no-fat milk

270 g (9½ oz/1 cup) apple purée

300 g (10½ oz) carrots, coarsely grated

nutrition per slice

Energy **1070 kJ (256 Cal)** Fat **6.4 g** Saturated fat **1.7 g** Protein **7.4 g** Carbohydrate **40 g** Fibre **4.9 g** Cholesterol **32 mg** Sodium **57 mg**

Ricotta topping

185 g (6½ oz/¾ cup) low-fat ricotta cheese

30 g (1 oz/¼ cup) icing (confectioners') sugar

1½ tsp grated lemon zest

15 g (½ oz/¼ cup) shredded coconut, lightly toasted

Prep time 20 minutes

Cooking time 1½ hours

Makes 12 slices

1 Preheat the oven to 180°C (350°F/Gas 4). Lightly grease a 21 x 11 cm (8¼ x 4¼ in) loaf (bar) tin and line the base with baking paper.

2 Sift the flours, bicarbonate of soda and spices into a large bowl. Return the husks to the bowl. Stir in the oat bran, sugar and sultanas. Combine the eggs, oil, milk and apple purée in a large bowl. Stir the egg mixture into the flour mixture, then stir in the carrot.

3 Spoon into the prepared tin and bake for 1¼ hours, or until a skewer comes out clean and the cake comes away slightly from the sides. Cover with foil if browning too much. Leave for 15 minutes, then turn out onto a wire rack.

4 To make the ricotta topping, beat ricotta, icing sugar and lemon zest together until smooth. Spread over the cooled cake and sprinkle over the toasted coconut.

Some websites with useful information

AUSTRALIA
Go Grains
www.gograins.com.au
Contains lots of information about the health benefits
of wholegrains and legumes.

The Cancer Council of Australia
www.cancer.org.au

The Gut Foundation
www.gutfoundation.com

Dietitians Association of Australia
www.daa.asn.au
At this site you'll find healthy eating advice, and can search
for an accredited practising dietitian in your area.

The Healthy Eating Club
www.healthyeatingclub.org
Provides information about nutrition and healthy eating.

UNITED KINGDOM
Cancer Research UK
www.cancerresearchuk.org

The British Dietetic Association
www.bda.uk.com

USA

National Digestive Diseases Information Clearinghouse (NDDIC)
www.digestive.niddk.nih.gov
Has information on digestive diseases such as constipation,
irritable bowel syndrome (IBS) and diverticulosis.

National Cancer Institute
www.cancer.gov
This website contains lots of information about various cancers,
including colon cancer.

American Dietetic Association
www.eatright.org

OTHER USEFUL WEBSITES

Irritable Bowel Syndrome Self Help and Support Group
www.ibsgroup.org

About Irritable Bowel Syndrome (IBS)
www.aboutibs.org

Glycaemic Index (GI) and GI Database
www.glycemicindex.com

Shepherd Works
www.shepherdworks.com.au
Provides information about diets low in fermentable oligosaccharides,
disaccharides, monosaccharides and polyols (FODMAPs) and their use
in IBS.

Index